Practical Pharmaceu

Other Examination Preparation Books Published by Petroc Press:

Obtainable from all good booksellers or, in case of difficulty, from Plymbridge Distributors Limited, Plymbridge House, Estover Road, PLYMOUTH, Devon PL6 7PZ

Tel.   01752–202300
FAX   01752–202333

Practical Pharmaceutical Calculations

M. C. Bonner

Lecturer in Pharmaceutical Technology
School of Pharmacy
University of Bradford, W. Yorkshire

D. J. Wright

Lecturer in Pharmacy Practice
School of Pharmacy
University of Bradford, W. Yorkshire

B. George

Teacher Practitioner
Leeds General Infirmary/School of Pharmacy
University of Bradford, W. Yorkshire

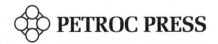 PETROC PRESS

Petroc Press, an imprint of LibraPharm Limited

Distributors
Plymbridge Distributors Limited, Plymbridge House, Estover Road,
Plymouth PL6 7PZ, UK

First edition 1999
Reprinted (with corrections) 2000, 2001

Published in the United Kingdom by
LibraPharm Limited
Gemini House
162 Craven Road
NEWBURY
Berks
RG14 5NR
UK

A catalogue record for this book is available from the British Library

ISBN 1 900603 57 8

Printed and bound in the United Kingdom by
MPG Books Limited, Bodmin, Cornwall PL31 1EG

Contents

Preface

The majority of health-care professionals will be carrying out pharmaceutical calculations on a daily basis. Errors in calculations, such as the volume of a mixture necessary to provide a certain dosage, or of the amount of an additive to an i.v. infusion, can have serious, and possibly fatal, consequences.

It is obviously important that all health-care professionals should have a good grasp of the fundamentals of practical pharmaceutical calculations. The book starts by introducing the reader to simple units of measurements and expressions of concentration, and leads on to a demonstration of how simple calculations can be used to estimate individual patient dosages. The progression through the book is aided with the help of numerous examples and the provision of stepwise solutions. At the end of each chapter, self-assessment calculations are provided, which are designed be used to test the reader's understanding. Fully worked solutions to all self-assessment calculations are also provided. It is not an aim of the book to enable students to perform the advanced pharmacokinetic calculations that may occasionally be required and that are now frequently carried out with the aid of a computer.

This book has been written to ensure that health-care students have a clear understanding of the type of pharmaceutical calculations that occur in day-to-day practice. We hope that by working logically through the book, the reader will develop a competency in these calculations and an ability to carry them out when necessary.

Bradford, 1999   M.C.B.
D.W.
B.G.

1 Units of Measurement

By the end of this chapter, you should be able to:

- Give the units of mass, volume and drug amount commonly used in pharmacy
- Convert between larger and smaller units of mass, volume and drug amount

1.1 The Metric System

In the UK, the metric system (or, more correctly, SI) is now the system that is most commonly used for the expression of quantities in pharmacy. For a particular quantity, a base unit exists: the gram is the base unit of mass, the litre is the base unit of volume and the mole is the base unit for drug amount. Prefixes are used to indicate quantities greater or less than the base unit. Table 1.1 lists the prefixes most commonly used in pharmacy, and gives an example of each.

Table 1.1 Prefixes used in the metric system

Prefix	Denoting	Example
kilo	One thousand times greater than the base unit	kilogram
milli	One thousand times less than the base unit	millilitre
micro	One million times less than the base unit	micromole

1.2 The Units of Mass

The most commonly used units of mass are listed in Table 1.2.

Table 1.2 Units of mass

Unit	Abbreviated to	Equivalent to
1 kilogram	kg	1000 grams
1 gram	g	1000 milligrams
1 milligram	mg	1000 micrograms
1 microgram	μg or mcg	1000 nanograms

Masses greater or less than these amounts are rarely used in pharmacy. To convert from smaller units to larger ones (e.g. milligrams to grams, grams to kilograms) we need to divide by 1000. Conversely, to convert from larger units into smaller ones (e.g. kilograms to grams, grams to milligrams) we must multiply by 1000 (Figure 1.1).

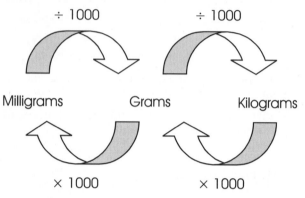

Figure 1.1   *Conversion between units of mass*

EXAMPLE 1.1

Add 0.00250 kg, 1750 mg, 2.50 g and 750,000 μg. Express your answer in grams.

Solution Steps

1. Convert each of the quantities to grams
2. Add the converted quantities together

0.00250 kg = (0.00250 × 1000) g	= 2.50 g
1750 mg = (1750 ÷ 1000) g	= 1.75 g
2.50 g	= 2.50 g
750,000 μg = (750,000 ÷ 1,000,000) g	= 0.75 g
Total mass	= 7.50 g

∴ **Answer = 7.50 g**

1.3   The Units of Volume

The base unit of volume is the litre (l, L, litre or ℓ). Table 1.3 gives the units of volume commonly used in pharmacy practice.

Table 1.3 *Units of volume used in pharmacy*

Unit	Abbreviated to	Equivalent to
1 litre	l, L, litre or ℓ	1000 millilitres
1 millilitre	ml	1000 microlitres

To convert volumes from litres into millilitres, we must multiply by 1000, and to convert volumes from millilitres into litres, we must divide by 1000 (Figure 1.2).

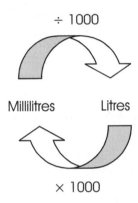

Figure 1.2 *Converting between units of volume*

EXAMPLE 1.2

Add 3 litre, 1150 ml and 0.75 litre. Give the total volume in millilitres

Solution Steps

1. Convert each of the quantities to millilitres
2. Add the converted quantities together

3 litres = (3 × 1000) ml	= 3000 ml
1150 ml	= 1150 ml
0.75 litre = (0.75 × 1000) ml	= 750 ml
Total volume	= 4900 ml

∴ **Answer = 4900 ml**

EXAMPLE 1.3

A patient is prescribed 10 ml of a mixture to be taken four times a day. How

*much of the mixture (in litres) is required to give the patient 30 days'
supply?*

Solution Steps

1. Calculate how much the patient takes each day
2. Calculate how much the patient then needs for 30 days
3. Convert this figure from millilitres to litres

<pre>
Each day the patient takes 10 ml × 4   =   40 ml
For 30 days the patient needs 40 ml × 30   = 1200 ml
1200 ml = (1200 ÷ 1000) litre   = 1.2 litre
</pre>

∴ **Answer = 1.2 litre**

1.4   Units of Drug Amount

The base unit for an amount of drug is the mole. One mole is the
amount of substance containing 6.02×10^{23} of its component
formula units (i.e. atoms, molecules or ions). The number of moles
of a drug may easily be expressed as a mass since a mole of a drug
weighs, in grams, the same as the relative molecular mass (R.M.M.)
of the substance. Thus, for example, one mole of potassium
chloride (R.M.M. = 74.5) weighs 74.5 g. Table 1.4 shows the units
of drug amount commonly used in pharmacy.

Table 1.4   *Units of drug amount*

Unit	Abbreviated to	Equivalent to
mole	mol	1000 millimoles
millimole	mmol	1000 micromoles

Figure 1.3 shows the conversion between moles and millimoles,
and their conversion into units of mass.

EXAMPLE 1.4

*How many millimoles of potassium chloride (R.M.M. = 74.5) are present in
149 g of the substance?*

Solution Steps

1. Calculate the number of moles of the drug

2. Convert this into millimoles

74.5 g is the weight of 1 mole of potassium chloride
1 g is the weight of 1 ÷ 74.5 mol of potassium chloride
149 g is the weight of 149 ÷ 74.5 mol of potassium chloride = 2 mol
2 mol = (2 × 1000) mmol = 2000 mmol

∴ **Answer = 2000 mmol**

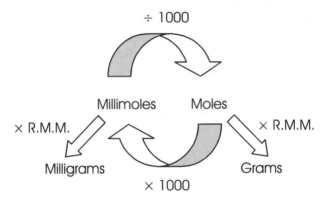

Figure 1.3   *Converting between units of drug amount*

1.5   Self-assessment

Now try the following self-assessment questions to ensure that you have understood this chapter.

Questions

1. Add 7 kg, 75 g and 750,000 mcg. Give your answer in grams.
2. Add 0.04 litre, 20 ml and 200 µl. Give your answer in millilitres.
3. A doctor prescribes 250 mg of tetracycline to be taken four times a day for 20 days. Calculate the total weight of tetracycline to be taken by the patient.
4. A capsule contains the following ingredients. Calculate, in grams, the amount of each ingredient required to manufacture 10,000 capsules:

Chlorpheniramine maleate   4 mg
Phenylpropanolamine hydrochloride   50 mg

5. A transdermal patch contains 8 mg of oestradiol. How many grams of oestradiol are required to make 50,000 patches?

6. An inhaler delivers 50 µg of salmeterol in each inhalation, and contains 200 metered inhalations. How many milligrams of salmeterol are present in the inhaler?

7. A patient is prescribed 15 ml of a mixture to be taken twice daily for 14 days. How much of the mixture should be supplied?

8. Sodium bicarbonate capsules each contain 500 mg of the compound. If a patient takes eight of these in a day, how many millimoles of sodium bicarbonate has the patient taken? (R.M.M. of sodium bicarbonate = 84.)

9. An intravenous infusion contains 30 mmol of sodium chloride. What is the mass of sodium chloride (in grams) contained in the infusion? (R.M.M. of sodium chloride = 58.5.)

10. An effervescent tablet for oral rehydration contains 117 mg of sodium chloride and 186 mg of potassium chloride. How many millimoles of *chloride* are contained in one tablet? (R.M.M. of sodium chloride (NaCl) = 58.5, R.M.M. of potassium chloride (KCl) = 74.5.)

2 Understanding Concentrations

By the end of this chapter you should:

- Be familiar with four different ways of expressing concentration – quantity per volume, percentage concentrations, ratios and parts.

- Understand the terms % w/v, % w/w and % v/v

- Know how to interpret a ratio expression of concentration

- Know how to interpret a parts expression of concentration

- Be able to convert between expressions of concentration

2.1 Expressions of Concentration

The vast majority of the pharmaceutical preparations used in the UK contain an active ingredient (drug) dissolved or dispersed in a solvent or diluent. Various expressions may be used to define the concentration of a drug in a preparation and a knowledge of these is essential in the practice of pharmacy. Additionally, the understanding of expressions of concentration is also important when examining clinical laboratory test results, as biochemical results may be given in a variety of ways. In this chapter, we will consider four different ways of expressing concentrations:

1. Quantity per volume
2. Percentage concentrations
3. Parts
4. Ratios

2.2 Quantity per Volume

Quantity per volume expressions are used to give the concentration of drugs in solution and also for clinical laboratory test results. A quantity-per-volume expression gives the amount or weight of drug (in terms of moles or grams, respectively) in a volume of solution. For example, a 9 g/l solution of sodium chloride means that 9 g of sodium chloride are dissolved in 1 litre of solution. A 1 mmol solution of sodium chloride contains 1 mmol (equivalent to 0.058 g) of the compound dissolved in 1 litre of solution.

EXAMPLE 2.1

What weight of sodium bicarbonate (in grams) is required to make 200 ml of a 6 g/l solution?

Solution Steps

1. Look at the concentration expression and work out how much is contained in 1 ml of solution
2. Calculate how much is required to make 200 ml of solution

   6 g/l means that 6 g of sodium bicarbonate must be dissolved in 1 litre (1000 ml) of solution

   So, 6 ÷ 1000 g of sodium bicarbonate must be dissolved in 1 ml of solution

   So, (6 ÷ 1000) × 200 g of sodium bicarbonate must be dissolved in 200 ml of solution = 1.2 g

EXAMPLE 2.2

A patient has a serum potassium level of 4 mmol/l. (a) How many millimoles of potassium are present in a 20 ml sample of the patient's serum? (b) How many milligrams of potassium are present in this sample? (R.M.M. of potassium = 39.)

Solution Steps (a)

1. Look at the concentration expression and calculate how many millimoles are present in 1 ml of serum
2. Calculate how many millimoles are present in 20 ml of serum

   4 mmol/l means that 4 mmol of potassium are present in 1 litre of serum

   So 4 ÷ 1000 mmol of potassium are present in 1 ml of serum

   Therefore (4 × 20) ÷ 1000 mmol of potassium are present in 20 ml of serum = 80 ÷ 1000 mmol = 0.08 mmol

Solution Steps (b)

1. Convert the number of millimoles to milligrams by multiplying by the R.M.M. (see Chapter 1)

1 mmol of potassium weighs 39 mg
0.08 mmol of potassium weigh 0.08 × 39 mg = 3.12 mg
0.08 mmol of potassium are present in 20 ml of serum
So, 3.12 mg of potassium are present in 20 ml of serum

2.3   Percentage Concentrations

Percentages may be used to express drug concentration in both liquid and solid dosage forms. A percentage concentration denotes the number of parts of a drug (either as grams or milligrams) in 100 parts of the dosage form. Three different percentage concentrations are commonly used, and their use depends on the nature of the product.

% w/v

This is the percentage weight in volume, used to express the weight of a solid in 100 ml of a liquid product. For example, a 1% w/v solution of sodium chloride in water denotes that 1 g of sodium chloride is contained in 100 ml of solution. To make this solution, 1 g of sodium chloride would be dissolved in a small volume of water, and the solution made up to 100 ml with water.

% w/w

This is the percentage weight in weight, used to express the weight of a solid, or occasionally a liquid, in 100 g of a solid product. For example, a 1% w/w hydrocortisone ointment denotes that 1 g of hydrocortisone is contained in 100 g of the final ointment. To make this product, 1 g of hydrocortisone would be mixed with a small weight of the ointment base and then the product would be made up to 100 g with further ointment base.

% v/v

This is the percentage volume in volume, used to express the volume of a liquid in 100 ml of a liquid product. For example, an emulsion containing 50% v/v liquid paraffin denotes that 50 ml of liquid paraffin are contained in 100 ml of the final emulsion.

EXAMPLE 2.3

A mouthwash contains 0.1% w/v chlorhexidine gluconate. How much chlorhexidine gluconate is contained in 250 ml of the mouthwash?

Solution Steps

1. Look at the concentration expression and determine how much drug is contained in 1 ml of the product
2. Calculate how much drug would therefore be contained in 250 ml of the product

   0.1% w/v denotes that 100 ml of the mouthwash contains 0.1 g of chlorhexidine gluconate
   So, 1 ml of the mouthwash contains 0.1 ÷ 100 g of chlorhexidine gluconate
   Therefore 250 ml of the mouthwash contains (0.1 ÷ 100) × 250 g of chlorhexidine gluconate = 0.25 g

EXAMPLE 2.4

What weight of miconazole is required to make 40 g of a cream containing 2% w/w of the drug?

Solution Steps

1. Look at the concentration expression and determine how much drug is contained in 1 g of the product
2. Calculate how much drug would therefore be contained in 40 g of the product

   2% w/w denotes that 100 g of the cream must contain 2 g of miconazole
   So, 1 g of the cream must contain 2 ÷ 100 g of miconazole
   Therefore 40 g of the cream must contain (2 ÷ 100) × 40 g of miconazole = 0.8 g

EXAMPLE 2.5

How much arachis oil is required to make 300 ml of an emulsion containing 30% v/v of arachis oil?

Solution Steps

1. Look at the concentration expression and determine how much arachis oil is contained in 1 ml of the product
2. Calculate how much arachis oil would therefore be contained in 300 ml of the product

   30% v/v denotes that 100 ml of the emulsion contains 30 ml of arachis oil
   So, 1 ml of the emulsion contains 30 ÷ 100 ml of arachis oil
   Therefore 300 ml of the emulsion contains (30 ÷ 100) × 300 ml of arachis oil = 90 ml

2.4   Ratio Concentrations

A ratio concentration is most commonly used to express the concentration of very dilute solutions. It expresses the number of parts (usually millilitres) of a solvent within which one part of the drug is dissolved or dispersed. Thus, a 1:5000 solution of a drug indicates that 1 g of the drug is dissolved in 5000 ml (5 litre) of solution.

EXAMPLE 2.6

How many milligrams of adrenaline are contained in 10 ml of a 1:10,000 solution of the drug?

Solution Steps

1. Convert the ratio to a quantity per volume expression
2. Calculate how much adrenaline is present in 1 ml of the solution
3. Calculate how much adrenaline is present in 10 ml of solution

   A 1:10,000 solution denotes that 1 g of adrenaline is dissolved in 10,000 ml of the solution
   So, 1 ml of the solution will contain 1 ÷ 10,000 g of adrenaline
   Therefore 10 ml of the solution will contain (1 ÷ 10,000) × 10 g of adrenaline = 0.001 g = 1 mg

2.5   Parts as Expressions of Concentration

This method of expressing concentrations is similar to ratio expressions except that the convention is to replace the ratio symbol with the word 'in'. Thus, a 1:1000 solution becomes a 1 in 1000, but the meaning is unchanged, i.e. 1 g of a drug dissolved in 1000 ml of a solution.

EXAMPLE 2.7

A 10 ml ampoule of a 1 in 200,000 solution of bupivacaine hydrochloride is administered to a patient. How many milligrams of bupivacaine hydrochloride does the patient receive?

Solution Steps

1. Convert the parts expression to a quantity per volume expression
2. Calculate how much bupivacaine hydrochloride is present in

   1 ml of the solution
3. Calculate how much bupivacaine hydrochloride is present in
   10 ml of solution

   A 1 in 200,000 solution denotes that 1 g of bupivacaine
      hydrochloride is dissolved in 200,000 ml of the solution
   So, 1 ml of the solution will contain 1 ÷ 200,000 g of bupiva-
      caine hydrochloride
   Therefore 10 ml of the solution will contain (1 ÷ 200,000) ×
      10 g of bupivacaine hydrochloride = 0.00005 g = 0.05 mg

2.6   Converting Between Expressions of Concentration

It is frequently necessary to convert between the various expressions of concentration. In order to do this, you should ensure that
you understand what is meant by each of the expressions of
concentration described previously.

EXAMPLE 2.8

*A solution contains 10 mg of drug in 5 ml of solution. Express this as a ratio
concentration.*

Solution Steps

1. Determine what concentration expression is required
2. As a ratio concentration is required, determine what volume
   of solution would contain 1 g of drug
3. Express this as a ratio

   10 mg of the drug is contained in 5 ml of the solution
   So, 1 mg of the drug is contained in 5 ÷ 10 ml of the solution
   Therefore 1 g of the drug is contained in (5 × 1000) ÷ 10 ml of
      the solution = 5000 ÷ 10 ml = 500 ml
   Therefore we have a 1:500 solution.

2.7   Self-assessment

Now try the following self-assessment questions to ensure that you
have understood this chapter.

Questions

1. A patient is prescribed a suspension containing 2 mg/ml of a drug. The directions are for the patient to take 10 ml of the suspension three times a day for one week. How many milligrams of the drug will the patient receive?

2. A patient dissolves two tablets, each containing 300 mg of aspirin, in 120 ml of water. What is the aspirin concentration (% w/v) of the solution?

3. How many grams of an antibiotic are required to prepare 50 ml of a 0.25% w/v solution of the antibiotic?

4. A liniment contains 5% v/v methyl salicylate. How much methyl salicylate is required to make 550 ml of the liniment?

5. How much hydrocortisone is present in 120 g of a cream containing 0.5% w/w hydrocortisone?

6. Sodium chloride infusion 0.9% w/v is used widely for electrolyte replacement. Express this concentration of sodium chloride in mmol/l. (R.M.M. of sodium chloride = 58.5.)

7. What volume of a 1:20,000 solution of adrenaline would contain 50 mg of the drug?

8. What is the % w/v concentration of a 1000 mmol solution of sodium bicarbonate? (R.M.M. of sodium bicarbonate = 84.)

9. A patient uses 200 ml of a 1:8000 solution of an antiseptic, daily, for seven days. How many grams of the antiseptic have been used?

10. You are provided with a powdered drug which contains 5% w/w moisture. What weight of the powder do you need to make 5 litre of an aqueous solution with a concentration of 4% w/v of the *anhydrous* drug?

3 Formulae for Extemporaneous Dispensing

By the end of this chapter you should be able to:

- Use a reference source formula to calculate quantities of each ingredient required to make a given amount of a pharmaceutical product
- Correctly interpret formulae where ingredient quantities are listed as parts or percentages

3.1 Reference Source Formulae

When a pharmaceutical product is to be prepared extemporaneously, a reference formula is usually required. These formulae can be found in the pharmaceutical reference sources, such as the *British Pharmacopoeia* or the *Pharmaceutical Codex*. A reference formula lists the ingredients of the preparation and the quantities of each required to make a certain weight or volume of it, depending on whether the preparation is a solid or a liquid. Frequently, the weight or volume of the preparation given in the reference formula will not be the same as that which must be prepared, in which case the quantities of each ingredient must be increased or reduced.

EXAMPLE 3.1

You are asked to prepare 300 ml of single strength chloroform water. The formula is given below.

Concentrated chloroform water   25 ml
Purified water   to 1000 ml

Solution Steps

1. As this is a liquid preparation, calculate how much of each component is required to make 1 ml of the product
2. Calculate, therefore, how much is required to make 300 ml of the product

Conc. chloriform water:

25 ml	25 ÷ 1000 ml	(25 ÷ 1000) × 300 ml	7.5 ml

Purified water:

to 1000 ml	to 1 ml	to 300 ml	to 300 ml

EXAMPLE 3.2

You are required to prepare 3500 g Zinc Cream BP. The formula is given below:

Zinc oxide	320 g
Calcium hydroxide	0.45 g
Oleic acid	5 ml
Arachis oil	320 ml
Wool fat	80 g
Purified water to produce	1000 g

Solution Steps

1. As this is a solid preparation, calculate how much of each component is required to make 1 g of the product
2. Calculate, therefore, how much is required to make 3500 g of the product

Zinc oxide:

320 g	320 ÷ 1000 g	(320 ÷ 1000) × 3500 g	1120 g

Calcium hydroxide:

0.45 g	0.45 ÷ 1000 g	(0.45 ÷ 1000) × 3500 g	1.57 g

Oleic acid:

5 ml	5 ÷ 1000 ml	(5 ÷ 1000) × 3500 ml	17.5 ml

Arachis oil:

320 ml	320 ÷ 1000 ml	(320 ÷ 1000) × 3500 ml	1120 ml

Wool fat:

80 g	80 ÷ 1000 g	(80 ÷ 1000) × 3500 g	280 g

Purified water:

to 1000 g	to 1 g	to 3500 g	to 3500 g

In the above two examples, the final line of the reference formula indicates that the product is to be made up to a certain weight or volume. However, this may not always be the case. Consider the formula for Hydrous Ointment BP in Example 3.3. The total weight of the ingredients is 1000 g, so the quantities of each ingredient must be scaled up or down, based upon how much of the product is required.

EXAMPLE 3.3

You are required to dispense 50 g of Hydrous Ointment BP. The formula is given below:

Wool alcohols ointment	500 g
Phenoxyethanol	10 g
Dried magnesium sulphate	5 g
Purified water	485 g

Solution Steps

1. Add together the quantities of each ingredient
2. Divide the quantity of each ingredient by this sum to find how much of each ingredient would be required to make 1 g of the product
3. Calculate the amounts required for 50 g

Total weight of the ingredients is 1000 g. Therefore:

Wool alcohols ointment:
  500 g   500 ÷ 1000 g   (500 ÷ 1000) × 50 g   25 g
Phenoxyethanol:
  10 g   10 ÷ 1000 g   (10 ÷ 1000) × 50 g   0.5 g
Dried magnesium sulphate:
  5 g   5 ÷ 1000 g   (5 ÷ 1000) × 50 g   0.25 g
Purified water:
  485 g   485 ÷ 1000 g   (485 ÷ 1000) × 50 g   24.25 g
Total weight:
  1000 g   1 g   50 g   50 g

3.2   Formulae in Parts or Percentages

Occasionally, the respective amounts of the ingredients are listed as either parts or percentages. This type of formula is usually written by a prescriber requesting 'special' ointments or creams.

EXAMPLE 3.4

Prepare 30 g of the following ointment:

Hydrocortisone ointment	25%
White soft paraffin	50%
Liquid paraffin	25%

Solution Steps

1. Work out the quantities of each ingredient that would be required to make 100 g of the product – these will be the same as the percentages

2. Calculate the amounts required for 30 g

Hydrocortisone ointment	25%	25 g	(25 ÷ 100) × 30 g	7.5 g
White soft paraffin	50%	50 g	(50 ÷ 100) × 30 g	15 g
Liquid paraffin	25%	25 g	(25 ÷ 100) × 30 g	7.5 g
Total weight		100 g		30 g	30 g

EXAMPLE 3.5

Prepare 400 g of the following cream:

Betamethasone cream	1 part
Aqueous cream	3 parts

Solution Steps

1. Sum the total number of parts
2. Divide the number of parts of each ingredient by this sum to obtain a fraction
3. Multiply this fraction by the required weight of the product to find the weight of each ingredient required

Total number of parts = 4
Required weight of Betamethasone cream = ¼ × 400 = 100 g
Required weight of Aqueous cream = ¾ × 400 = 300 g

3.3   Self-assessment

Now try the following self-assessment questions to ensure that you have understood this chapter.

Questions

1. Prepare 250 ml of Acid Gentian Mixture BP

Acid Gentian Mixture BP

Concentrated compound gentian infusion	100 ml
Dilute hydrochloric acid	50 ml
Double strength chloroform water	500 ml
Water	to 1000 ml

2. Prepare 150 ml of Potassium Citrate Mixture BP

   Potassium Citrate Mixture BP

Potassium citrate	300 g
Citric acid monohydrate	50 g
Lemon spirit	5 ml
Quillaia tincture	10 ml
Syrup	250 ml
Double strength chloroform water	300 ml
Water	to 1000 ml

3. Prepare 300 ml of Chloral Elixir Paed. BP

   Chloral Elixir Paed. BP

Chloral hydrate	200 mg
Water	0.1 ml
Blackcurrant syrup	1 ml
Syrup	to 5 ml

4. Prepare 200 ml of Paediatric Ferrous Sulphate Mixture BP

   Paediatric Ferrous Sulphate Mixture BP

Ferrous sulphate	60 mg
Ascorbic acid	10 mg
Orange syrup	0.5 ml
Double strength chloroform water	2.5 ml
Water	to 5 ml

5. What quantities of each ingredient are required to prepare 50 g of Coal Tar and Zinc Ointment BP?

   Coal Tar and Zinc Ointment BP

Strong coal tar solution	100 g
Zinc oxide	300 g
Yellow soft paraffin	600 g

6. What quantity of each ingredient is required to prepare 600 g of Zinc and Salicylic Acid Paste BP?

Zinc and Salicylic Acid Paste BP

Zinc oxide	24%
Salicylic acid	2%
Starch	24%
White soft paraffin	50%

7. Prepare 5000 ml of Magnesium Hydroxide Mixture BP

Magnesium Hydroxide Mixture BP

Magnesium sulphate	47.5 g
Sodium hydroxide	15 g
Light Magnesium Oxide	52.5 g
Chloroform	2.5 ml
Water	to 1000 ml

8. Prepare 30 g of the following ointment:

| Fluocinolone acetonide cream | 10% |
| Aqueous cream | to 100% |

9. Prepare 75 g of the following cream:

| Betamethasone cream | 1 part |
| Aqueous cream | 4 parts |

10. Prepare 80 g of the following ointment:

| Dithranol ointment | 1 part |
| White soft paraffin | to 4 parts |

(*Caution:* Read the second line of the formula carefully)

4 Dilution, Mixing and Incorporation

By the end of this chapter you should be able to:

- Carry out calculations involving the dilution of solutions and solid preparations
- Carry out calculations involving the mixing of solutions and solid preparations
- Carry out calculations involving the incorporation of medicaments into solid preparations

4.1 Dilution of Solutions

The dilution of solutions is one of the most frequently carried out calculations in pharmacy. A stock solution, or concentrate, must often be diluted to a particular strength for patient use. This type of calculation is particularly common for antiseptic and disinfectant preparations. In a dilution, the weight of the active ingredient will stay the same throughout – therefore a simple formula for these calculations may be derived:

Mass of active before dilution = Mass of active after dilution

However   Conc. of active = Mass of active ÷ Volume of solution
Therefore   Mass of active = Conc. of active × Volume of solution
Hence   (Before dilution) Conc. of active (C_1) × Volume of solution (V_1) = Conc. of active (C_2) × Volume of solution (V_2) (after dilution)

Abbreviating $C_1 \times V_1 = C_2 \times V_2$

For this equation to hold, both concentrations must be expressed in the same units and both volumes must also be expressed in the same units.

EXAMPLE 4.1

How many millilitres of a 10% w/v solution of an antiseptic must be used to make 4 litres of a 0.25% w/v solution?

Solution Steps

1. Fill in the appropriate values in the equation

$$C_1 \times V_1 = C_2 \times V_2$$

2. Rearrange the equation to find the unknown (V_1)

$C_1 = 10\%$ w/v
$V_1 = ?$
$C_2 = 0.25\%$ w/v
$V_2 = 4$ litre

$10 \times V_1 = 0.25 \times 4$
Thus, $V_1 = (0.25 \times 4) \div 10 = 0.1$ litres $= 100$ ml

EXAMPLE 4.2

How many millilitres of water must be ADDED to 250 ml of an 18% w/v stock solution of sodium chloride to prepare a 0.9% w/v sodium chloride solution?

Solution Steps

1. Fill in the appropriate values in the equation

$$C_1 \times V_1 = C_2 \times V_2$$

2. Rearrange the equation to find the unknown (V_1)
3. As we need to find out how much water must be ADDED to carry out the dilution, subtract 250 ml from V_2

$C_1 = 18\%$ w/v
$V_1 = 250$ ml
$C_2 = 0.9\%$ w/v
$V_2 = ?$

$18 \times 250 = 0.9 \times V_2$
Therefore $V_2 = (18 \times 250) \div 0.9 = 5000$ ml
However, to carry out the dilution, 5000 ml – 250 ml must be added = 4750 ml

EXAMPLE 4.3

How many millilitres of a 1:5000 solution of phenylmercuric nitrate can be made from 250 ml of a 0.2% w/v solution of the compound?

Solution Steps

1. Make the expressions of concentration similar
2. Fill in the appropriate values in the equation

$$C_1 \times V_1 = C_2 \times V_2$$

3. Rearrange the equation to find the unknown (V_2)

A 1:5000 solution means that 1 g of the active is dissolved in 5000 ml

So, $1 \div 5000$ g is dissolved in 1 ml

Therefore $(1 \div 5000) \times 100$ g is dissolved in 100 ml = 0.02 g in 100 ml = 0.02% w/v

C_1 = 0.2% w/v
V_1 = 250 ml
C_2 = 0.02% w/v
V_2 = ?

$0.2 \times 250 = 0.02 \times V_2$
Therefore $V_2 = (0.2 \times 250) \div 0.02 = 2500$ ml

4.2 Dilution of Solid Preparations

Occasionally, a prescriber may request the dilution of active ingredients in a solid preparation. As the weight of active ingredient in the preparation will remain the same during the dilution, the following formula should be used.

(Before dilution) Conc. of active (% w/w) × Total mass of product = Conc. of active (% w/w) × Total mass of product (after dilution)

Abbreviating $\qquad C_1 \times M_1 = C_2 \times M_2$

EXAMPLE 4.4

You are supplied with 50 g of salicylic acid ointment 2% w/w. What weight of emulsifying ointment (diluent) should be added to reduce the concentration of salicylic acid to 0.5% w/w?

Solution Steps

1. Fill in the appropriate values in the equation

$$C_1 \times M_1 = C_2 \times M_2$$

2. Rearrange the equation to find the unknown (M_2)
3. As we need to find out how much emulsifying ointment must be added to carry out the dilution, subtract 50 g from M_2

$C_1 = 2\%$ w/w
$M_1 = 50\,g$
$C_2 = 0.5\%$ w/w
$M_2 = ?$

$2 \times 50 = 0.5 \times M_2$
Therefore $M_2 = (2 \times 50) \div 0.5 = 200\,g$
However, to carry out the dilution 200 g – 50 g must be added = 150 g

4.3   Mixing of Solutions

If two or more solutions of the same active ingredient are mixed, the final concentration of the ingredient may be calculated readily.

EXAMPLE 4.5

What is the concentration of dextrose in a solution prepared by mixing 200 ml of 10% w/v dextrose, 50 ml of 20% w/v dextrose, and 100 ml of 5% w/v dextrose?

Solution Steps

1. Calculate the weight of dextrose in each of the solutions to be mixed
2. Calculate the total volume of the mixture produced
3. From these, calculate the concentration of dextrose in the mixture

10% w/v dextrose will contain 10 g dextrose in 100 ml of solution
Hence 1 ml of solution contains 10 ÷ 100 g of dextrose
So, 200 ml of solution contains (10 ÷ 100) × 200 g of dextrose = 20 g of dextrose
20% w/v dextrose will contain 20 g dextrose in 100 ml of solution

Therefore 1 ml of solution contains 20 ÷ 100 g of dextrose

So, 50 ml of solution contains (20 ÷ 1000) × 50 g of dextrose = 10 g of dextrose

5% w/v dextrose will contain 5 g of dextrose in 100 ml of solution

So, 5 g of dextrose are present in this solution

The total weight of dextrose = 20 g + 10 g + 5 g = 35 g

The total volume of mixture = 200 ml + 50 ml + 100 ml = 350 ml

Hence the mixture contains 35 g of dextrose dissolved in 350 ml of solution

Thus, 1 ml of solution contains (35 ÷ 350) g of dextrose

So, 100 ml of solution contains (35 ÷ 350) × 100 g of dextrose = 10 g

The mixture therefore contains 10% w/v dextrose

A more common problem in pharmacy is one where a solution of a particular concentration is required, and it must be produced from a mixture of two other solutions.

EXAMPLE 4.6

You are presented with a 500 ml infusion bag containing 5% w/v dextrose and a number of ampoules containing 15% w/v potassium chloride. A prescriber requests that sufficient potassium chloride is added to the infusion bag so that it will contain 0.3% w/v potassium chloride.

Solution Steps

1. Let the weight of potassium chloride required to be added = x g
2. Construct an equation where the final weight of potassium chloride in the bag divided by its final volume is = (0.3 ÷ 100)
3. Solve for x
4. Calculate the volume of 15% w/v potassium chloride which must contain x g

The solution that must be produced is to contain 0.3 g of potassium chloride in each 100 ml of solution. Irrespective of the final volume of the solution, this concentration must be obtained

Let the weight of potassium chloride to be added to the bag be x g

The following equation can be constructed:

$$\frac{\text{Final weight of drug}}{\text{Final volume of solution}} = \frac{0.3}{100}$$

This is equivalent to:

$$\frac{\text{Initial weight of drug } + \text{ added weight of drug}}{\text{Initial volume of solution } + \text{ added volume of solution}} = \frac{0.3}{100}$$

Initial weight of drug in the bag = 0
Added weight of drug = x g
Initial volume of solution = 500 ml
Added volume of solution = $(100 \div 15)x$ ml
Since 15 g of potassium chloride are dissolved in 100 ml of the
  solution
1 g of potassium chloride is dissolved in $100 \div 15$ ml of the
  solution
Therefore x g of potassium chloride is dissolved in
  $(100 \div 15)x$ ml of the solution
Substituting into the equation:

$$\frac{0 + x}{500 + \dfrac{100x}{15}} = \frac{0.3}{100}$$

Cross-multiplying:

$$0.3\left(500 + \frac{100x}{15}\right) = 100(0 + x)$$

thus $150 + 2x = 100x$
Rearranging, $98x = 150$ and hence $x = 1.53$ g
1.53 g of potassium chloride are dissolved in $(100 \div 15) \times$
  1.53 ml of the 15% w/v solution = 10.2 ml
Hence 10.2 ml of the 15% w/v potassium chloride must be
  added to the infusion bag

4.4 Incorporation of Medicaments into Solid Preparations

If we need to increase the concentration of an active ingredient in a
cream or ointment by the addition of pure extra ingredient, then a
calculation similar to Example 4.6 must be carried out. The next
example will illustrate the point.

EXAMPLE 4.7

*What weight of coal tar extract must be added to 100 g of a cream containing
1% w/w coal tar extract to produce a cream containing 5% coal tar extract?*

Solution Steps

1. Let the weight of coal tar extract to be added = x g
2. Construct an equation where the final weight of coal tar in the cream divided by the final weight of the cream is $5 \div 100$
3. Solve for x

The cream that must be produced is to contain 5 g of coal tar extract in each 100 g of cream. Irrespective of the final weight of the cream, this concentration must be obtained

Let the weight of coal tar extract to be added = x g

The following equation can then be constructed:

$$\frac{\text{Final weight of drug}}{\text{Final weight of cream}} = \frac{5}{100}$$

In this case, this is equivalent to:

$$\frac{\text{Initial weight of drug + added weight of drug}}{\text{Initial weight of cream + added weight of drug}} = \frac{5}{100}$$

Initial weight of drug = 1 g (since we have 100 g of a 1% w/w cream)

Added weight of drug = x g

Initial weight of cream = 100 g

$$\frac{1+x}{100+x} = \frac{5}{100}$$

Cross-multiplying:

$$100(1 + x) = 5(100 + x)$$
$$100 + 100x = 500 + 5x$$

Rearranging, $95x = 400$

and hence $x = 4.21$ g

4.5 Self-assessment

Now try the following self-assessment questions to ensure that you have understood this chapter.

Questions

1. How many millilitres of a 0.2% w/v solution of an antiseptic must be used to prepare 1 litre of a 1:5000 solution?
2. What volume of a 1:5000 solution of cetrimide can be made from 100 ml of a 4% solution of cetrimide?
3. A patient is directed to use 50 ml of a 1:10,000 solution of potassium permanganate solution twice a day for five days. You have in stock a 2% w/v solution of the compound. How much of the concentrate will you require to dispense the prescription?
4. How many millilitres of water must be *added* to 50 ml of 13% w/v aluminium acetate solution to prepare a 0.65% w/v solution?
5. How many grams of emulsifying ointment must be *added* to 200 g of 5% w/w calamine in emulsifying ointment, in order to reduce the calamine concentration to 2% w/w?
6. You have an infusion solution – volume 1 litre – of 0.3% w/v potassium chloride and a number of ampoules containing 25% w/v dextrose. What volume of the 25% w/v solution of dextrose must be added to the infusion bag to produce a concentration of 5% w/v dextrose?
7. A prescriber requests that sufficient potassium chloride is added to 500 ml of a 0.9% w/v sodium chloride infusion to give a final concentration of 40 mmol/l potassium. What volume of a 15% w/v potassium chloride solution should be added to the infusion? (R.M.M. of potassium = 39.)
8. A cream (weight 30 g) contains 0.1% w/w dithranol. What weight of dithranol powder should be added to increase the concentration to 1% w/w?
9. Salicylic acid ointment contains 2% w/w salicylic acid. What weight of salicylic acid powder should be added to 50 g of the ointment to produce a 10% w/w ointment?
10. A cream contains 10% w/w coal tar solution. What weight of coal tar solution should be incorporated into this cream to produce 30 g of cream containing 12% w/w coal tar solution?

5 Dose Calculations

By the end of this chapter you should be able to:

- Calculate doses for adult patients based on their actual and ideal body weight, and their surface area
- Calculate doses for paediatric patients based on their actual body weight and their surface area
- Calculate infusion rates for intravenous drips and syringe pumps

5.1 Dosage Calculations

There are many drugs for which there are no standard doses, and for these drugs calculation of the dose required is dependent on a patient characteristic, such as body weight or surface area.

EXAMPLE 5.1

What dose of salbutamol syrup would your recommend for a 10-year-old child, weight 30 kg, when the recommended dosage is 100 mcg/kg?

In this example the dose would be 30 kg × 100 mcg/kg = 3000 mcg = 3 mg

EXAMPLE 5.2

What dose of vincristine is required in a 92 kg patient with a body surface area (BSA) of 2.0 m^2 and a recommended dosage of 1.4 mg/m^2?

In this example the dose would be 2.0 m^2 × 1.4 mg/m^2 = 2.8 mg

Table 5.1 summarises the most common dosage units based upon a patient's weight or surface area.

Table 5.1   *Patient characteristics and corresponding dose units*

Characteristics	Dose units	Abbreviated to
Weight	Grams per kilogram	g/kg
	Milligrams per kilogram	mg/kg
	Micrograms per kilogram	mcg/kg
	Units of drug per kilogram	U/kg
Body surface area	Grams per square metre of surface area	g/m^2
	Milligrams per square metre of surface area	mg/m^2
	Micrograms per square metre of surface area	mcg/m^2
	Units of drug per square metre of surface area	U/m^2

In the first example the patient's actual body weight (ABW) was used. In some instances it is more appropriate to use the patient's ideal body weight (IBW). Calculation of ideal body weight is necessary for adult patients whose body weight is more than either 30% above, or 30% below, the average adult weight of 70 kg (i.e. for very obese or emaciated patients).

Where drugs are predominantly distributed in the lean tissues, e.g. digoxin, either the ABW or IBW are used depending on which is the lower.

Calculation of Ideal Body Weight

Ideal body weight is calculated from the patient's height H (cm) using the following equations:

$$\text{Males:} \quad \text{IBW} = (0.9 \times H) - 88$$

$$\text{Females:} \quad \text{IBW} = (0.9 \times H) - 92$$

Estimation of Body Surface Area

In the second example, body surface area (BSA) was used and this is usually obtained from the patient's height and actual body weight. The patient's surface area can be determined from these two parameters by using one of two following methods:

- Nomograms for calculating BSA are provided in standard medical texts[1]. The same nomograms can be used for adults and children who are more than one year old. Infants (less than one year old) generally have their own nomogram.

- The formula[2] for estimating BSA, provided below, is suitable for use with adults and children and is considered to be more accurate than the nomogram method. Height H (cm) and weight W (kg) are used to determine the BSA (m^2).

$$\text{Surface area formula: } BSA = \sqrt{\frac{H \times W}{3600}}$$

EXAMPLE 5.3

The dosage of the chemotherapeutic agent cyclophosphamide can be expressed in mg/m^2 in some regimens and in mg/kg in other regimens. If the doses required are either 60 mg/kg or 800 mg/m^2 for a male adult patient who weighs 92 kg and measures 1.6 m, give three possible doses to be administered based on ABW, IBW and BSA.

Solution Steps

1. Calculate the patient's IBW
2. Calculate the patient's BSA
3. Calculate the dose using ABW, IBW and BSA

$$ABW = 92 \, kg$$
$$IBW = 0.9H - 88 = (0.9 \times 160) - 88 = 56 \, kg$$

$$BSA = \sqrt{\frac{H \times W}{3600}} = \sqrt{\frac{160 \times 92}{3600}} = 2.022 \, m^2$$

$$\begin{aligned}
\text{Dose based on ABW} &= 92 \times 60 &&= 5520 \, mg \\
\text{Dose based on IBW} &= 56 \times 60 &&= 3360 \, mg \\
\text{Dose based on BSA} &= 2.02 \times 800 &&= 1617.6 \, mg
\end{aligned}$$

5.2 Dose Calculations for Paediatrics

Paediatric doses are usually calculated on the basis of weight or surface area in a similar manner to the adult dose examples presented in Table 5.1. As stated earlier, infants under one year old have a separate nomogram for the determination of surface area.

If specific paediatric doses cannot be found, however, the percentage method of dose calculation is sometimes used. Table 5.2 shows the relationship between the average weight for a child's age and the percentage of the adult dose that the child should receive.

Table 5.2 *Percentage method for calculating doses[3]*

Age	Mean weight for age (kg)	Percentage of adult dose
Neonate (full term)	3.5	12.5
2 months	4.5	15
4 months	6.5	20
1 year	10	25
3 years	15	33.3
7 years	23	50
10 years	30	60
12 years	39	75
14 years	50	80
16 years	58	90
Adult	68	100

EXAMPLE 5.4

A 3-year-old child of average weight is prescribed a drug for which there is no known paediatric dose. The adult dose of the drug is 600 mg daily. How much could you give the child using the percentage method of dose calculation (to the nearest milligram)?

Solution Steps

1. Establish what percentage of the adult dose the child should receive
2. Establish the normal adult dose
3. Divide the quoted percentage by 100 and multiply by the adult dose

A 3-year old of average weight should receive 33.3% of the adult dose

The normal adult dose is 600 mg daily

Therefore the dose for the child = $(33.3 \div 100) \times 600 = 199.8$ (or 200) mg daily

5.3 Infusion Rates

Some drugs, e.g. frusemide, phenytoin, potassium chloride and vancomycin, have maximum rates over which they can be infused. Infusion rates are usually limited owing to toxic effects, which may occur if these drugs are given too rapidly.

Doses for drugs such as dopamine and dobutamine used in acute situations are often expressed in quantity of drug to be delivered per kilogram of body weight per minute. It is important, therefore, to understand how to calculate infusion rates and give accurate advice about how these drugs should be delivered.

EXAMPLE 5.5

A dose of 4 mcg/kg/minute of dopamine is required to be infused into a 70 kg patient over 2 h. What volume of dopamine 0.16% w/v infusion is required?

Solution Steps

1. Calculate the total amount of dopamine required
2. Identify the amount of dopamine in 100 ml of infusion
3. Calculate the volume of infusion required to provide the total amount of dopamine required

The patient requires 4 mcg/kg/min × 70 kg × 120 min = 33,600 mcg = 33.6 mg

In 100 ml of 0.16% w/v infusion there will be 0.16 g = 160 mg

Therefore the volume of infusion required is

$$\frac{33.6 \text{ mg}}{160 \text{ mg}} \times 100 \text{ ml} = 21 \text{ ml}$$

EXAMPLE 5.6

A dopamine infusion is set up for a 60 kg female, to deliver 2.5 mcg/kg/min. The syringe contains 200 mg of dopamine in 50 ml of normal saline. What should the infusion rate be in millilitres/hour?

Solution Steps

1. Calculate the dose required in terms of milligrams/hour
2. Establish the number of milligrams/millilitre in the dopamine infusion
3. Divide the dose in milligrams/hour by the number of milligrams of dopamine in each millilitre of infusion to give the infusion rate in millilitres/hour required

Dose required is 2.5 mcg/kg/min = 2.5 mcg × 60 kg = 150 mcg/min = 150 mcg × 60 min = 9000 mcg/h (or 9 mg/h)

Infusion contains 200 mg in 50 ml = 200/50 mg in 1 ml = 4 mg/ml

Therefore the rate required = 9 mg/h ÷ 4 mg/ml = 2.25 ml/h

Intravenous infusions which do not require as much accuracy in their delivery (e.g. routine fluid replacement or blood transfusion) are administered using standard giving sets and require calculation of drop rates. Drop volumes supplied by standard giving sets are given in Table 5.3.

Table 5.3   *Drop volumes for standard giving sets*

Adult	Paediatric	Blood
1 ml = 20 drops	1 ml = 60 drops	1 ml = 15 drops

EXAMPLE 5.7

An adult giving set with fixed drop size and adjustable flow is being used to deliver 1 litre of normal saline over 12 hours. What should the drop rate be set at, in drops/minute?

Solution Steps

1. Establish how many drops are in 1 ml
2. Calculate how many millilitres need to be delivered every minute to give 1 litre in 12 hours
3. Multiply the number of millilitres per minute by the number of drops in each millitre

   Adult giving set delivers 20 drops per millilitre
   1 litre in 12 h = (1000 ml ÷ 12) in 1 h = 83.3 ml in 1 h
   83.3 ml in 1 h = (83.3 ml ÷ 60) in 1 min = 1.4 ml in 1 min
   Therefore 1.4 ml/min = 1.4 × 20 drops/min = 28 drops/min

5.4   Self-assessment

Now try the following self-assessment questions to ensure that you have understood this chapter.

Questions

1. Phenytoin can be given orally as a 3–4 mg/kg daily dose. What dose should be given to an 80 kg female who is 1.5 m tall in order to give 3 mg/kg based on:

   (a) Actual body weight?
   (b) Ideal body weight?

2. The adult dose of drug x is 600 mg, but there is no recommended paediatric dose. Based on Table 5.2 in Chapter 5, what dose would you advise for a two-month-old child, weighing 4.6 kg, of drug x?
3. Methotrexate can be prescribed based on weight or surface area. Using an appropriate equation, calculate the dose required for a 65 kg male (1.7 m in height) based on a pre-

scribed dose of 500 mg/m^2

4. A patient with DVT is prescribed heparin infusion of 2000 U/h. If the nurse has used PumpHep (1000 units/millilitre of infusion) to fill a 50 ml syringe:

   (a) At what rate should the infusion be delivered (in milli-litres/hour)?
   (b) How long will it take, theoretically, for the syringe to deliver the infusion?

5. A patient is prescribed 250 mg frusemide IV. This should not be given more rapidly than 4 mg/min.

   (a) What is the minimum time over which this dose can be given?
   (b) Rather than administering the drug neat, a pharmacist advises that the frusemide dose is dissolved in 50 ml of normal saline. At what rate (millilitres/minute) should the drug be administered?

6. A patient is prescribed 80 mmol of potassium, which is to be given using two litres of fluid and at a rate of 20 mmol/h. If a normal giving set delivers approximately 20 drops per millilitre, calculate the drip rate required, in drops per minute, to administer the potassium.

7. A paediatric giving set (1 ml = 60 drops) is being used to administer 250 ml of saline over 24 h. What should the drop rate be set at, in drops/minute?

8. A diabetic patient is being controlled by using an IV sliding scale. A syringe pump containing 75 U of soluble insulin in 50 ml of saline is available. The patient's blood glucose is measured every hour and the insulin dose is adjusted according to the scale below.

Fingerprick glucose (mmol/l)	IV soluble insulin (units/h)
< 2	None – give 50 ml 50% w/v dextrose
2.0–6.4	0.5
6.5–8.9	1.0
9.0–10.9	2.0
11–16.9	3.0
17–28	4.0
> 28	8.0

   If the patient's blood glucose is currently 12.3 mmol/l, what pump rate should be used (in millilitres/hour)?

9. A syringe pump on the ward is delivering dopamine infusion

200 mg/50 ml at a rate of 3.1 ml/h to a 70 kg male. What dose (in mcg/kg/min) is he receiving (to the nearest whole number)?

10. A dobutamine infusion is running at 2.4 ml/h for a 65 kg female; the syringe contains 250 mg dobutamine in 50 ml normal saline. What increase is necessary in the infusion rate to increase the dose delivered by 0.5 mcg/kg/min?

References

1. *The Smith Kline and French Clinical Pharmacy Handbook* (1989). SKF Laboratories.
2. Mosteller, R. D. (1987). Simplified calculation of body-surface area. *NEJM*, **317**, 1098.
3. *Guy's and Lewisham and St Thomas' Hospitals' Paediatric Formulary*. 3rd edn, C. S. Printers Ltd.

6 Clinical Pharmacokinetics

By the end of this chapter you should be able to:

- Estimate loading dosages
- Estimate maintenance dosages
- Determine renal function from serum creatinine concentrations

6.1 Definition of Terms

Pharmacokinetic calculations are used to increase the likelihood of obtaining drug serum concentrations within a required range. These calculations invariably require the use of equations and therefore it is appropriate to define the common terminology.

Therapeutic Window

The therapeutic window is the serum concentration range within which a drug is most likely to be clinically effective and least likely to cause unwanted side-effects. A serum concentration within the 'therapeutic window' does not, however, demonstrate clinical effectiveness. Clinical indicators are always necessary to determine the effectiveness of therapy.

The majority of drugs have a wide therapeutic window and consequently close monitoring of the drug's serum concentration is not clinically justified. Drugs such as digoxin, theophylline, gentamicin, carbamazepine and phenytoin all have narrow therapeutic windows (Table 6.1) and hence for patients prescribed these drugs it is important to individualise dosages very carefully. Local biochemistry laboratories may use differing values, depending on the standardisation of the equipment.

Table 6.1   *Therapeutic windows for regularly prescribed drugs*

Drug	Serum concentration range
Digoxin	1–2 mcg/l
Theophylline	10–20 mg/l*
Phenytoin	10–20 mg/l*
Carbamazepine	4–12 mg/l
Gentamicin	4–8 mg/l (peak)

*Theophylline and phenytoin can be effective from 5 mg/l

Bioavailability

Bioavailability (F) is the fraction of the drug that reaches the systemic circulation and is expressed as a number from 0 to 1. Drugs that are metabolised in the gut or liver are poorly absorbed and will have reduced bioavailability. The effect of metabolism in the liver is generally described as the *first pass effect*. A large first pass effect will invariably produce a low oral bioavailability. Similarly, different formulations and routes of administration can significantly affect bioavailability. It is generally accepted that drugs that are parenterally administered, e.g. gentamicin, have a bioavailability of 1. The approximate bioavailabilities of regularly used formulations of drugs with narrow therapeutic windows are outlined in Table 6.2.

Table 6.2   *Approximate bioavailability of regularly prescribed formulations*

Drug and formulation	F
Digoxin tablets	0.7
Digoxin elixir	0.77
Phenytoin preparations*	1
Carbamazepine tablets (Tegretol)	1.0
Carbamazepine s/r tablets (Tegretol Retard)	0.85
Aminophylline s/r tablets†	1
Theophylline s/r tablets and capsules	1

*Phenytoin capsules and injections consist of the sodium salt, and the salt fraction (S) must be taken into account when determining the amount of phenytoin absorbed. The S value is 0.92 for both preparations.
†Aminophylline is a theophylline salt and consequently the S value must be taken into account when determining the amount of theophylline absorbed. Approximately 80% by weight of aminophylline is theophylline and hence any aminophylline dose must be multiplied by 0.8 to determine the amount of theophylline reaching the systemic circulation.

In Summary

Amount of drug reaching systemic circulation = Bioavailability × Salt fraction × Dose administered

i.e. $= F \times S \times$ Dose

EXAMPLE 6.1

What dose of carbamazepine slow-release tablets would be required if a patient were to be changed from a dose of 1000 mg of carbamazepine normal-release tablets, to ensure that the same amount of drug was delivered to the systemic circulation?

Solution Steps

1. Calculate the amount of carbamazepine systemically absorbed from normal release tablets
2. Calculate the dose of the new formulation required to deliver the same amount of carbamazepine to the systemic circulation

   The dose of carbamazepine systemically absorbed by the patient from the normal release tablets is:

   $F \times S \times$ Oral dose = Amount systemically absorbed
   $1 \times 1 \times$ 1000 mg = 1000 mg absorbed

   Therefore 1000 mg must be systemically absorbed from the slow-release tablets
   Rearranging the above equation gives:

   $$\text{Oral dose} = \frac{\text{Amount systemically absorbed}}{F \times S}$$

   $$= \frac{1000 \text{ mg}}{0.85 \times 1} = 1176.4 \text{ mg}$$

   In practice, the prescribed dose would be 1200 mg because 200 mg is the lowest available dosage of slow-release carbamazepine.

Volume of Distribution

When a drug has been delivered into the systemic circulation its distribution around the body depends on its lipid and water solubility. Hence the final drug concentration in different tissues will vary. The serum concentration of a drug is most commonly quoted.

The volume of distribution (V_d), used in pharmacokinetic calculations, is the theoretical volume that would be needed to distribute a drug, if it was found at the same concentration throughout the body as that measured in the serum. For example, if a patient has a measured drug serum concentration (C) of 15 mg/l and we know that 300 mg had been systemically absorbed, then the volume of distribution would be 20 litre, i.e. 20 litre of serum would be needed to distribute the dose (300 mg ÷ 15 mg/l = 20 litre). So,

$$\text{Volume of distribution} = \frac{\text{Amount of drug systemically absorbed}}{\text{Serum concentration}}$$

But as we know that:

Amount systemically absorbed = $F \times S \times$ Dose

$$\text{Volume of distribution} = \frac{F \times S \times \text{Dose}}{C}$$

The time at which a serum concentration is measured is important if the drug does not immediately distribute itself between the serum and body tissues. If a drug is initially predominantly distributed in the serum then a serum concentration taken too soon after administration will produce an artificially high result and the V_d will be calculated as being smaller than the actual value. Drugs undergoing this type of distribution, e.g. digoxin, are described as distributing via a two-compartment model. A digoxin serum concentration should be measured within 6 h after dosing to calculate accurately V_d.

The population average volumes of distribution per kilogram of actual body weight (ABW), excepting digoxin, for drugs with a narrow therapeutic index, is provided in Table 6.3.

Table 6.3 *Population volumes of distribution for regularly prescribed drugs*

Drug	Volume of distribution (litre/kg)
Digoxin	7.3*
Theophylline	0.5
Phenytoin	0.65
Carbamazepine	1.4
Gentamicin	0.25

*Based upon ideal or actual body weight, whichever is lower

Elimination Half-life

This is the time it takes for a drug serum concentration to reduce by half after all the drug has been delivered into the systemic circulation. Table 6.4 gives the average elimination half-life ($T_{0.5}$) of commonly prescribed drugs with a narrow therapeutic window. This information is especially useful for determining how long to withdraw a drug for, when an overdose is detected. For example, in the case of a drug with $T_{0.5} = 12\,h$ it would take 24 h for the serum concentration to reduce from 20 mg/l to 5 mg/l. This is because after 12 h the serum concentration will be 10 mg/l and after a further 12 h it will be 5 mg/l.

Table 6.4   *Approximate $T_{0.5}$ values for regularly prescribed drugs*

Drug	$T_{0.5}$
Digoxin	48 h
Theophylline	8 h
Phenytoin	22 h*
Carbamazepine	30–35 h

*The half-life of phenytoin is dependent on the serum concentration, and consequently this value can vary.

Clearance

Clearance is the volume of serum that is cleared of a drug over a set period of time, and is usually expressed in litres per hour. Clearance does not tell you the exact amount of drug cleared, because this is dependent on the drug's serum concentration.

EXAMPLE 6.2

If a drug has a clearance of 2 litre/h, how much will be removed from the body in 24 h if:

(a) The serum concentration is 4 mg/l?
(b) The serum concentration is 1 mg/l?

Solution Steps

1. Multiply the volume cleared per hour by the serum concentration to determine the total amount of drug cleared in one hour
2. Multiply the total amount of drug cleared in one hour by 24 hours

(a) If 2 litre of serum are cleared each hour and every litre of serum has 4 mg of drug in it, then 8 mg will be cleared each hour.

Amount of drug removed in 24 h will be 8 mg/h × 24 h = 192 mg

(b) If 2 litre of serum are cleared each hour and every litre has 1 mg of drug in it, then 2 mg will be cleared each hour.

Amount of drug removed in 24 h will be 2 mg/h × 24 h = 48 mg.

Table 6.5 summarises the average clearance values for drugs with small therapeutic windows. Individual patient clearances can be calculated from the population values provided in Table 6.5, by multiplying by the actual body weight of the patient. The clearance of digoxin, phenytoin and gentamicin are dependent on other factors, and the calculation of these is provided below.

Table 6.5 *Population 'clearance' for theophylline and carbamazepine*

Drug	Clearance (litre/h/kg)
Theophylline	0.04
Carbamazepine	0.064

Because digoxin and gentamicin are predominantly removed by the kidneys, prior calculation of renal function is necessary to estimate the drug clearance.

Creatinine Clearance

Creatinine clearance (Cl_{cr}) is the most practical and accurate measure of renal function and is most easily determined using serum creatinine concentrations. Because these are not independent of age, sex or weight, these must also be taken into account in the calculations. The equations for calculating creatinine clearance (measured in millilitres per minute) in both males and females are provided below:

Males

$$Cl_{cr} \text{ (ml/min)} = \frac{1.23(140 - \text{Age}) \times \text{Weight (kg)}}{\text{Serum creatinine } (\mu\text{mol/litre})}$$

Females

$$Cl_{cr} \ (ml/min) \ = \ \frac{1.04(140 - Age) \times Weight \ (kg)}{Serum \ creatinine \ (\mu mol/litre)}$$

Because creatinine is a by-product of muscle metabolism, either the patient's ideal body weight (IBW, see Chapter 5) or ABW, whichever is lower, should be used.

Once a creatinine clearance has been calculated, then the degree of renal impairment can be estimated using the following guidelines:

Cl_{cr} < 10 ml/min	Severe renal impairment
Cl_{cr} 10–20 ml/min	Moderate renal impairment
Cl_{cr} > 20 ml/min and < 50 ml/min	Mild renal impairment

EXAMPLE 6.3

Calculate the renal function of Mrs AS, a 75-year-old patient, who is 1.6 m tall, weighs 65 kg and has a measured serum creatinine of 130 μmol/l.

Solution Steps

1. Calculate the patient's ideal body weight (IBW)
2. Place either the IBW or ABW, whichever is the lowest, into the equation for determining creatinine clearance for females
3. Use the clearance value obtained to determine the degree of renal impairment

Firstly, we need to calculate the IBW for a female

IBW (female) = $0.9H - 92$ = $(0.9 \times 160 \, cm) - 92$ = 52 kg
ABW = 65 kg

The weight to be used in the equation is therefore 52 kg.

$$Cl_{cr} \ (females) \ = \ \frac{1.04(140 - Age) \times Weight \ (kg)}{Serum \ creatinine \ (\mu mol/litre)} \ (ml/min)$$

$$Cl_{cr} \ (females) \ = \ \frac{1.04(140 - 75) \times 52}{130 \mu mol/litre} \ (ml/min)$$

$$Cl_{cr} = 27 \, ml/min$$

We can therefore assume that this patient has mild renal impairment.

Digoxin Clearance

Digoxin clearance is calculated by summing the renal and metabolic clearance of the drug. Renal clearance of digoxin is approximately equal to creatinine clearance, and metabolic clearance can be estimated, although it is dependent on whether the patient has congestive heart failure. The presence of congestive heart failure can reduce metabolic and renal clearance of digoxin by 50% and 10%, respectively.

In a patient without heart failure:

$$\text{Digoxin clearance (ml/min)} = (0.8 \times \text{Weight (kg)}) + \text{Cl}_{cr}$$

In a patient with congestive heart failure:

$$\text{Digoxin clearance (ml/min)} = (0.33 \times \text{Weight (kg)}) + (0.9 \times \text{Cl}_{cr})$$

EXAMPLE 6.4

Estimate the digoxin clearance of Mrs AS, who has an estimated creatinine clearance of 27 ml/min and weighs 65 kg. Assume that Mrs AS does not have congestive heart failure.

Solution Step

1. Place the values provided into the equation for digoxin clearance for a patient without congestive heart failure

$$\begin{aligned}
\text{Digoxin clearance (ml/min)} &= (0.8 \times \text{Weight (kg)}) + \text{Cl}_{cr} \\
&= (0.8 \times 65) + 27 \\
&= 79 \, \text{ml/min}
\end{aligned}$$

Gentamicin Clearance

Gentamicin is almost entirely renally excreted, consequently creatinine clearance and gentamicin clearance are the same, unless renal function is markedly diminished. In this instance the non-renal clearance of 0.0021 litre/h/kg is used to estimate gentamicin clearance.

Phenytoin Clearance

Phenytoin metabolism is capacity limited, meaning that when the amount of phenytoin entering the body passes a certain point, the metabolism of the drug cannot increase accordingly. Consequently, increases in dosage can lead to disproportionate increases in serum concentration.

The metabolism of phenytoin follows the pattern proposed by Michaelis and Menten, and the variables V_m and K_m are used to describe phenytoin pharmacokinetics.

- V_m is the maximum metabolic capacity (mg/day)
- K_m is the plasma concentration at which the rate of metabolism is half the maximum (mg/l)

Using the Michaelis Menten model, phenytoin clearance is calculated from the equation:

$$\text{Clearance of phenytoin (Cl}_{\text{Phenytoin}}) = \frac{V_m}{K_m + \text{Serum concentration (mg/l)}}$$

EXAMPLE 6.5

Assuming that V_m is 7 mg/kg/day and K_m is 4 mg/l, calculate the phenytoin clearance in a 60 kg patient with a serum concentration of 15 mg/l.

Solution Step

1. Place the values provided into the equation for the clearance of phenytoin

$$\text{Clearance of phenytoin (Cl}_{\text{Phenytoin}}) = \frac{V_m}{K_m + \text{Serum concentration (mg/l)}}$$

$$= \frac{7 \, \text{mg/kg/day} \times 60 \, \text{kg}}{4 \, \text{mg/l} + 15 \, \text{mg/l}}$$

$$= 22.1 \, \text{litre/day}$$

In practice, K_m can usually be assumed to be 4 mg/l, and for initial estimates, V_m may be taken as 7 mg/kg/day. However, the value for V_m should always be revised after the first serum concentration has been measured. In order to calculate a revised V_m, the following equation should be used:

$$V_m = \frac{S \times F \times \text{Daily dose (mg)} \times (K_m + \text{Serum concentration})}{\text{Serum concentration}}$$

This equation can also be rearranged to calculate maintenance dosages:

$$\text{Maintenance dose (mg)} = \frac{V_m \times \text{Serum concentration}}{S \times F \times (K_m + \text{Serum concentration})}$$

EXAMPLE 6.6

Estimate the phenytoin maintenance dosage for a 60 kg patient requiring a serum concentration of 15 mg/l. (Assuming that K_m is 4 mg/l and that V_m is 7 mg/kg/day, and that the patient is to receive capsules.)

Solution Step

1. Place the values provided into the equation for estimating phenytoin maintenance dosages

   From previous information we know that:

   Bioavailability F = 1
   Salt fraction S = 0.92
   K_m = 4 mg/l
   V_m = 7 mg/kg/day

   $$\text{Maintenance dose (mg)} = \frac{V_m \times \text{Serum concentration}}{S \times F \times (K_m + \text{Serum concentration})}$$

   $$= \frac{(7 \times 60) \times 15}{1 \times 0.92 \times (4 + 15)}$$

   = 360 mg phenytoin sodium capsules
   (350 mg in practice)

EXAMPLE 6.7

After prescribing 350 mg of phenytoin sodium capsules for 5 days to a 60 kg patient, the measured serum concentration is 10 mg/l. What dose would be necessary to provide a serum concentration of 15 mg/l?

Solution Steps

1. Determine V_m using the serum concentration and dose provided
2. Estimate the phenytoin maintenance dosage with the new V_m

   From previous information we know that:

   Bioavailability F = 1
   Salt fraction S = 0.92
   K_m = 4 mg/l

$$\text{Maintenance dose (mg)} = \frac{V_m \times \text{Serum concentration}}{S \times F \times (K_m + \text{Serum concentration})}$$

Firstly, we need to calculate V_m

$$V_m = \frac{0.92 \times 1 \times (350 \text{ mg}) \times (4 + 10)}{10}$$

$$V_m = 450.8 \text{ mg / day}$$

$$\text{Maintenance dose (mg)} = \frac{V_m \times \text{Serum concentration}}{S \times F \times (K_m + \text{Serum concentration})}$$

$$= \frac{450.8 \times 15}{1 \times 0.92 \times (4 + 15)}$$

$$= 386.8 \text{ mg phenytoin sodium capsules}$$
$$\text{(400 mg in practice)}$$

6.2   Loading Dose

If we can estimate a patient's volume of distribution and know the target concentration required, it is possible to estimate an individual patient's loading dose. The amount of drug in the body will be the target serum concentration multiplied by the volume of distribution. The loading dose will then be equal to the amount of drug in the body divided by the bioavailability and salt fraction of the equation used.

$$\text{Amount of drug in the body} = \text{Target conc. } (C) \times \text{Volume of distribution } (V_d)$$

$$\text{Loading dose} = \frac{\text{Amount of drug in the body}}{\text{Bioavailability } (F) \times \text{Salt fraction } (S)}$$

Substituting:

$$\text{Loading dose} = \frac{C \times V_d}{F \times S}$$

EXAMPLE 6.8

It is decided that Mrs Jones requires Digoxin therapy. She is 60 kg in weight. What oral loading dose would you recommend?

Solution Steps

1. Calculate the patient's volume of distribution
2. Use the equation for loading dose to determine the required dosage

From previous information we know that:

F = 0.7
V_d = 7.3 litre/kg
C = 1.5 mcg/l

This patient's volume of distribution is therefore

$$7.3 \text{ litre/kg} \times 60 \text{ kg} = 438 \text{ litre}$$

$$\text{Loading dose} = \frac{C \times V_d}{F \times S}$$

$$= \frac{1.5 \text{ mcg/litre} \times 438 \text{ litre}}{0.7 \times 1}$$

$$= 938.6 \text{ mcg}$$

In practice, the prescriber would give 1000 mcg as an oral dose.

EXAMPLE 6.9

What dose of gentamicin would be required to achieve a target concentration of 6 mg/l in an 80 kg woman?

From previous information we know that:

F = 1
S = 1
V_d = 0.25 litre/kg
C = 6 mg/l

This patient's volume of distribution is therefore

$$0.25 \, \text{litre/kg} \times 80 \, \text{kg} = 20 \, \text{litre}$$

$$\text{Required dose} = \frac{V_\text{d} \times C}{F \times S}$$

$$= \frac{20 \, \text{litre} \times 6 \, \text{mg/l}}{1 \times 1}$$

$$= 120 \, \text{mg gentamicin}$$

One of the assumptions of using the above equation for estimating loading dosages is that, during the time taken for the drug to be systemically absorbed, there is very little elimination from the body. This assumption generally holds true if elimination of the drug is slow, i.e. it has a long half-life, or if its absorption is rapid. Because gentamicin has a relatively short half-life, the validity of the above equation is dependent on the rate of infusion. In general, if the infusion time is less than one quarter of the half-life (gentamicin $T_{0.5} = 2$–3 h) then the above equation can be used. Equations to determine the loading dose of gentamicin, which take into account elimination of the drug, are beyond the remit of this book.

6.3 Maintenance Dosages

The amount of drug required to keep a steady serum concentration is the maintenance dose. By multiplying the drug clearance by the required serum concentration we can calculate how the drug is removed, and therefore the amount required to replace it.

$$\text{Amount of drug removed} = V_\text{d} \times C$$

$$\text{Maintenance dose} = \frac{\text{Amount of drug removed}}{F \times S}$$

$$\text{Maintenance dose (mg/h)} = \frac{V_\text{d} \times C}{F \times S}$$

$$\text{Therefore maintenance dose every } \tau \text{ hours} = \frac{V_\text{d} \times C \times \tau}{F \times S}$$

EXAMPLE 6.10

What maintenance dose would you recommend, to be given every 6 h, if a drug has a clearance of 5 litre/h and a serum concentration of 15 mg/l? (Assume F = 1 and S = 1.)

Solution Step

1. Use the equation for maintenance dosage

$$\text{Maintenance dose} = \frac{\text{Clearance (litre/h)} \times \text{Concentration (mg/l)} \times \tau}{\text{Bioavailability } (F) \times \text{Salt fraction } (S)}$$

$$= \frac{5\,\text{litre/h} \times 15\,\text{mg/l} \times 6}{1 \times 1}$$

$$= 450\,\text{mg every 6 h}$$

EXAMPLE 6.11

Calculate the required daily digoxin maintenance dose for an 80 kg, 75-year-old male patient (1.9 m tall), with a serum creatinine of 130 μmol/l and no heart failure. The required serum concentration is 1.5 mcg/l.

Solution Steps

1. Calculate the patient's ideal body weight (IBW)
2. Determine the patient's renal function using either the IBW or ABW, whichever is the lowest
3. Calculate the patient's digoxin clearance
4. Calculate the required maintenance dose

From previous information we know that:

F = 0.7 for digoxin tablets
S = 1
C = 1.5 mcg/l
τ = 24 h

Firstly we need to calculate the patient's ideal body weight.

$$\text{IBW (male)} = 0.9H - 88 = 0.9\,(190) - 88 = 83\,\text{kg}$$

In this case the weight to be used is the patient's own weight. Next we need to determine the patient's renal function.

$$Cl_{cr} \text{ (Males)} = \frac{1.23(140 - \text{Age}) \times \text{Weight (kg)}}{\text{Serum creatinine } (\mu\text{mol/l})}$$

$$= \frac{1.23(140 - 75) \times 80}{130}$$

$$= 49.2\,\text{ml/min (mild renal impairment)}$$

Next we need to determine the digoxin clearance.

Digoxin clearance (ml/min) = (0.8 × Weight (kg)) + Cl_{cr}
$$= 64 + 49.2 = 113.2\,\text{ml/min} = 6.8\,\text{litre/h}$$

Finally, we can calculate the recommended maintenance dose.

$$\text{Maintenance dose} = \frac{V_d \times C \times \tau}{F \times S}$$

$$= \frac{6.8\,(\text{litre/h}) \times 1.5\,(\text{mcg/litre}) \times 24}{0.7 \times 1}$$

$$= 349.3\,\text{mcg daily}$$
$$(375\,\text{mcg in practice})$$

6.4 Self-assessment

Now try the following self-assessment questions to ensure that you have understood this chapter.

Questions

For each of the following questions, you may use the previously stated population values.

1. After giving a patient 1200 mg of carbamazepine tablets (normal release), a peak serum concentration of 12 mg/l was measured. Estimate the patient's volume of distribution.
2. 100 mcg of a new drug formulation was given to a patient and a total of 85 mcg was recovered in the urine. Calculate the bioavailability of the drug assuming that it is totally renally excreted.
3. A patient presents in casualty with a peak theophylline serum concentration of 30 mg/l. How long will it take for the serum concentration to reach 7.5 mg/l?
4. Estimate the renal impairment of a 55 kg, 80-year-old male (1.65 m tall) with a serum creatinine of 180 μmol/l.
5. What loading dose of IV digoxin would you recommend for a 60 kg patient requiring a serum concentration of 1.5 mcg/l?
6. What loading dose of IV aminophylline would you recommend for a 65 kg patient requiring a serum concentration of 10 mg/l?

7. Estimate the gentamicin serum concentration of a 70 kg patient that would be expected 1 h after a rapidly absorbed infusion of 100 mg had been started. Assume that there had been negligible elimination after 1 h.

8. What daily maintenance dose of digoxin would you recommend for a 75-year-old, 55 kg female (1.6 m tall) with congestive heart failure and a measured serum creatinine of 170 μmol/l?

9. A 55 kg patient prescribed 300 mg of phenytoin capsules daily has a measured serum concentration of 8 mg/l. What dosage of phenytoin would you recommend in order to obtain a serum concentration of 12 mg/l?

10. What twice-daily maintenance dose of carbamazepine (slow release tablets) would you recommend for a 70 kg male, if the target concentration was 10 mg/l?

7 Suppository Calculations

By the end of this chapter you should be able to:

- Calculate quantities of base and drug required for the preparation of theobroma oil and glycero-gelatin medicated suppositories

7.1 Suppositories

Suppositories are dosage forms prepared for drug delivery via the rectum. They consist of an active medicament dispersed throughout an inactive base. The bases used in these products can be broadly classified into two groups:

- Fatty bases. These may be of natural origin, such as theobroma oil (cocoa butter), or synthetic fats such as Witepsol.
- Hydrophilic bases. The most commonly used hydrophilic base is composed of a solid glycerol/gelatin mixture.

Displacement Values

Suppositories are prepared by dissolving or dispersing an active medicament in a molten base and pouring the mixture into a suppository mould. Suppository moulds are normally available in 1 g, 2 g and 4 g sizes – the approximate weights of the theobroma oil suppositories that are produced from them – although the volume of the suppository mould will be constant. However, because the density of the medicament may vary considerably from that of the base, the weight of the base required to make a suppository will vary depending on the medicament used. For example, 2 g of a medicament with twice the density of theobroma oil would occupy approximately the same volume as 1 g of the suppository base. The displacement values (DVs) of medicaments are required when calculating the weight of suppository base required to prepare medicated suppositories (Example 7.1). The displacement value of a medicament is the number of parts, by weight, of a medicament that will displace one part of suppository base (normally theobroma oil). Displacement values for various medicaments are given in the *Pharmaceutical Codex*.

(*Note:* The following examples take no account of preparation losses and it is normal practice to prepare for an excess quantity of suppositories.)

EXAMPLE 7.1

Calculate the quantities required to make 10 theobroma oil suppositories (2g mould) each containing 400mg of zinc oxide. (Displacement value = 4.7.)

Solution Steps

1. Calculate the total weight of zinc oxide required
2. Calculate what weight of base would be required to prepare 10 unmedicated suppositories
3. Determine what weight of base would be displaced by the medicament
4. Calculate, therefore, the weight of base required to prepare the medicated suppositories

   Total weight of zinc oxide required = 400 mg × 10 = 4 g
   Weight of base required for unmedicated suppositories = 2 g × 10 = 20 g

   As the displacement value of zinc oxide = 4.7, this means that 4.7 g of zinc oxide would displace 1 g of theobroma oil and 1 g of zinc oxide would displace 1 ÷ 4.7 g of theobroma oil
   Hence 4 g of zinc oxide will displace (4 × 1) ÷ 4.7 g of theobroma oil = 0.85 g
   Therefore the weight of base required to make medicated suppositories = 20 − 0.85 g = 19.15 g

Glycero-gelatin base has a density 1.2 times greater than theobroma oil, therefore a 1 g suppository mould will produce a 1 g theobroma oil suppository, but a 1.2 g glycero-gelatin suppository. This factor must be taken into account in displacement value calculations.

EXAMPLE 7.2

Calculate the quantities required to make six glycero-gelatin suppositories (4 g mould), each containing 100 mg aminophylline. (Displacement value = 1.3.)

Solution Steps

1. Calculate the total weight of aminophylline required
2. Calculate what weight of glycero-gelatin base would be required to prepare 10 unmedicated suppositories
3. Determine what weight of base would be displaced by the medicament
4. Calculate, therefore, the weight of base required to prepare the medicated suppositories

Total weight of aminophylline required = 100 mg × 6 = 600 mg or 0.6 g

Weight of base required for unmedicated suppositories = 4 g × 6 × 1.2 (to take account of the greater density of this base) = 28.8 g

Since the displacement value of aminophylline = 1.3, this means that 1.3 g of aminophylline displaces 1 g of theobroma oil

and therefore 1 g of aminophylline displaces 1 ÷ 1.3 g of theobroma oil

and 0.6 g of aminophylline displace (1 × 0.6) ÷ 1.3 g of theobroma oil = 0.46 g of theobroma oil

This means that the aminophylline would displace 0.46 g × 1.2 of the glycero-gelatin base = 0.55 g

Therefore the weight of base required to make medicated suppositories = 28.8 g – 0.55 g = 28.25 g

Medicaments Included as a % w/w

If a medicament is present in a suppository as a percentage w/w, then its displacement value is not required when calculating the respective amounts of medicament and base required to prepare the suppository.

EXAMPLE 7.3

What quantities are required to prepare in a 4 g mould eight theobroma oil suppositories each containing 1% w/w lignocaine hydrochloride?

Solution Steps

1. Calculate the total weight of the medicated suppositories

2. Calculate, therefore, the weight of the drug required (1% of the total weight)
3. Subtract the weight of the drug from the total weight of the suppositories to find the weight of the base required

Total weight of the suppositories = 32 g
Weight of drug required (1% w/w) = (32 × 1) ÷ 100 g = 0.32 g
Therefore weight of base required = 32 g – 0.32 g = 31.68 g

Again, if a glycero-gelatin base is used, the appropriate correction factor must be used, as a 1 g mould for a theobroma oil suppository will actually hold 1.2 g of glycero-gelatin base.

EXAMPLE 7.4

Prepare 12 glycero-gelatin suppositories, containing 0.5% w/w cinchocaine hydrochloride. Use a 2 g mould.

Solution Steps

1. Calculate the total weight of the medicated suppositories, allowing for the greater density of the glycero-gelatin base
2. Calculate the weight of the drug required
3. Subtract the weight of the drug from the total weight of the suppositories to determine the weight of the base required

Total weight of the suppositories = 12 × 2 g × 1.2 = 28.8 g
Weight of drug required = (28.8 g × 0.5) ÷ 100 = 0.144 g (or 144 mg)
Therefore weight of base required = 28.8 g – 0.144 g = 28.66 g

7.4   Self-assessment

Now try the following self-assessment questions to ensure that you have understood this chapter.

Questions

1. Prepare 14 theobroma oil suppositories (1 g mould) containing 2.5% w/w bismuth subgallate.
2. Prepare six theobroma oil suppositories (2 g mould) containing 10% w/w zinc oxide.
3. Six theobroma oil suppositories (2 g), each containing 125 mg of paracetamol, are to be prepared. The displacement value of

paracetamol is 1.5. What quantities of base and medicament are required?

4. You are asked to prepare 12 theobroma oil suppositories (2 g mould) each containing 300 mg of aspirin (DV = 1.1). What weights of base and medicament are required?

5. Prepare 10 theobroma oil suppositories, each containing 50 mg of bismuth subgallate (DV = 2.7). If a 2 g mould is used, what quantities of base and medicament are required?

6. A prescriber requests that eight glycero-gelatin suppositories be made, containing 1% w/w hydrocortisone acetate. If a 4 g mould is used, what quantities of base and medicament are needed?

7. Prepare six glycero-gelatin suppositories (in a 2 g mould) each containing 20 mg of morphine hydrochloride (DV = 1.6).

8. Ten glycero-gelatin suppositories, each containing 30 mg phenobarbitone sodium (displacement value 1.2), are to be prepared using a 1 g mould. What quantities of base and medicament are required?

9. Prepare 12 glycero-gelatin suppositories, in a 2 g mould, each containing 50 mg of diphenhydramine hydrochloride (DV = 1.3).

10. You are required to prepare 10 theobroma oil suppositories (2 g). Each suppository must contain 60 mg of bismuth subgallate (DV = 2.7) and 10 mg of hydrocortisone acetate (DV = 1.5). Calculate the weight of each medicament and of the theobroma oil required to prepare the suppositories.

(*Hint:* Calculate the weight of base displaced by each medicament and subtract both these from the weight of the unmedicated suppositories.)

Thus $\qquad \dfrac{150 \times 25}{100}$

Rearranging ... = 150 and hence = 1.53g

1.53g of potassium chloride are dissolved in (100×15) =

1.53 ml of the 15% w/v solution = 10.2 ml

Hence 10.2 ml of the 15% w/v potassium chloride must be added to the infusion bag

4.4 Incorporation of Medicaments into Solid Preparations

If we need to increase the concentration of an active ingredient in a cream or ointment by the addition of pure extra ingredient, then a calculation similar to example 4.6 must be carried out. The next example will illustrate the point.

EXAMPLE 4.7

What weight of coal tar extract must be added to 100g of a cream containing 15% w/w coal tar extract to produce a cream containing 25% coal tar extract?

Summary Test

Questions

1. Add 0.25 litre, 75 ml and 4000 µl. Give your answer in ml.
2. A patient is prescribed 5 ml of a mixture to be taken four times a day for seven days. How much of the mixture should be supplied?
3. An intravenous infusion contains 80 mmol of potassium chloride. What is the mass of potassium chloride (in grams) contained in the infusion? (R.M.M. of potassium chloride = 74.5.)
4. How much salicylic acid is present in 350 g of a cream containing 2% w/w salicylic acid?
5. What volume of a 1:10,000 solution of adrenaline would contain 20 mg of the drug?
6. A patient uses 50 ml of a 1:1000 solution of an antiseptic mouthwash, four times a day, for seven days. How many grams of the antiseptic have been used?
7. Prepare 500 ml of Chloral Elixir Paed. BP.

   Chloral Elixir Paed. BP:

Chloral hydrate	200 mg
Water	0.1 ml
Blackcurrant syrup	1 ml
Syrup	to 5 ml

8. What quantity of each ingredient is required to prepare 150 g of Coal Tar and Zinc Ointment BP?

   Coal Tar and Zinc Ointment BP:

Strong coal tar solution	100 g
Zinc oxide	300 g
Yellow soft paraffin	600 g

9. What quantity of each ingredient is required to prepare 400 g of Zinc and Salicylic acid Paste BP?

   Zinc and Salicylic acid Paste BP:

Zinc oxide	24%
Salicylic acid	2%
Starch	24%
White soft paraffin	50%

10. A patient is directed to use 20 ml of a 1:10,000 solution of potassium permanganate twice a day for 10 days. You have in stock a 4% w/v solution of the compound. How much of the concentrate will you require to dispense the prescription?

11. How many grams of emulsifying ointment must be *added* to 400 g of 2% w/w salicylic acid in emulsifying ointment, in order to reduce the salicylic acid concentration to 0.5% w/w?

12. A prescriber requests that sufficient dextrose be added to 500 ml of a 0.18% w/v sodium chloride infusion to give a final concentration of 4% w/v dextrose. What volume of a 40% w/w dextrose solution should be added to the infusion?

13. An ointment contains 1% w/w calamine. What weight of calamine powder should be added to 200 g of the ointment to produce a 5% w/w calamine ointment?

14. A patient is prescribed 5 mg bumetanide in 500 ml glucose 5% w/v, via IV infusion. This should not be given more rapidly than 100 mcg/min. At what rate (ml/min) should the drug be administered?

15. A syringe pump is delivering dopamine infusion 160 mg/50 ml at a rate of 5 ml/h to a 80 kg male. What dose (in mcg/kg/min) is he receiving?

16. Calculate the renal function of an 80-year-old female patient, who is 1.7 m tall, weighs 60 kg and has a measured serum creatinine of 170 μmol/l.

17. What loading dose would you recommend for an 80 kg, 1.8 m tall male patient requiring digoxin orally and a serum concentration of 1.2 mcg/l?

18. What daily maintenance dose of digoxin would you recommend for the same 80 kg, 1.8 m tall male patient (Question 17), with congestive heart failure, a creatinine clearance of 18 ml/min and a required serum concentration of 1.2 mcg/l?

19. Prepare 12 theobroma oil suppositories, each containing 100 mg of bismuth subgallate (DV = 2.7). If a 4 g mould is used, what quantities of base and medicament are required?

20. A prescriber requests that six glycero-gelatin suppositories be made, containing 0.5% w/w hydrocortisone acetate. If a 2 g mould is used, what quantities of base and medicament are needed?

Answers to the Self-assessment Questions

Chapter 1

1. 7 kg   = 7000 g
   75 g   = 75 g
   750,000 mcg = 750 mg   = 0.75 g
   Total weight   = 7075.75 g

2. 0.04 litre   = 40 ml
   20 ml   = 20 ml
   200 µl   = 0.2 ml
   Total volume   = 60.2 ml

3. Daily, the patient takes 4×250 mg tetracycline $= 1000$ mg $= 1$ g tetracycline. In 20 days, the patient takes 1 g $\times 20 = 20$ g tetracycline

4. Weight of chlorpheniramine maleate required:

   4 mg $\times 10,000 = 40,000$ mg $= 40$ g

   Weight of phenylpropanolamine hydrochloride required:

   50 mg $\times 10,000 = 500,000$ mg $= 500$ g

5. Weight of oestradiol required:

   8 mg $\times 50,000 = 400,000$ mg $= 400$ g

6. Weight of salmeterol in each inhaler:

   50 mcg $\times 200 = 10,000$ mcg $= 10$ mg

7. Daily, the patient takes 15 ml $\times 2 = 30$ ml

   In 14 days, the patient will take 30 ml $\times 14 = 420$ ml

8. Weight of sodium bicarbonate taken $= 500$ mg $\times 8 = 4000$ mg $= 4$ g

84 g of sodium bicarbonate is equivalent to 1 mol, or 1000 mmol
1 g of sodium bicarbonate is equivalent to 1000 ÷ 84 mmol
4 g of sodium bicarbonate is equivalent to (1000 ÷ 84) × 4 mmol = 47.6 mmol

9. 1 mol of sodium chloride weighs 58.5 g
1 mmol of sodium chloride weighs 58.5 mg
30 mmol of sodium chloride weighs 58.5 × 30 mg = 1755 mg = 1.75 g

10. 58.5 g of sodium chloride is equivalent to 1 mol
58.5 mg of sodium chloride is equivalent to 1 mmol
1 mg of sodium chloride is equivalent to 1 ÷ 58.5 mmol
117 mg of sodium chloride is equivalent to (1 ÷ 58.5) × 117 mmol = 2 mmol

74.5 g of potassium chloride is equivalent to 1 mol
74.5 mg of potassium chloride is equivalent to 1 mmol
1 mg of potassium chloride is equivalent 1 ÷ 74.5 mmol
186 mg of potassium chloride is equivalent to (1 ÷ 74.5) × 186 mmol = 2.5 mmol

1 mmol of sodium chloride provides 1 mmol of chloride
1 mmol of potassium chloride provides 1 mmol of chloride
Therefore the total amount of chloride = 2 + 2.5 mmol = 4.5 mmol

Chapter 2

1. Each dose contains 2 mg × 10 = 20 mg of drug
Daily, the patient takes 20 mg × 3 = 60 mg of drug
In one week, the patient takes 60 mg × 7 = 420 mg of drug

2. Weight of aspirin dissolved = 300 mg × 2 = 600 mg
600 mg of aspirin are dissolved in 120 ml water
0.6 g of aspirin are dissolved in 120 ml water
0.6 ÷ 120 g of aspirin are dissolved in 1 ml water
(0.6 ÷ 120) × 100 g of aspirin are dissolved in 100 ml water = 0.5 g
0.5 g of aspirin are dissolved in 100 ml water
Therefore the concentration of the solution is 0.5% w/v

3. 0.25 g of the antibiotic are dissolved in 100 ml of the solution
0.25 ÷ 100 g of the antibiotic are dissolved in 1 ml of the solution

(0.25 ÷ 100) × 50 g of the antibiotic are dissolved in 50 ml of solution = 0.125 g of the antibiotic are required.

4. 100 ml of the liniment contains 5 ml of methyl salicylate
   1 ml of the liniment contains 5 ÷ 100 ml of methyl salicylate
   550 ml of the liniment contains (5 × 550) ÷ 100 ml of methyl salicylate
   (5 × 550) ÷ 100 ml = 27.5 ml of methyl salicylate

5. 100 g of cream will contain 0.5 g hydrocortisone
   1 g of cream will contain 0.5 ÷ 100 g hydrocortisone
   120 g of cream will contain (0.5 ÷ 100) × 120 g hydrocortisone = 0.6 g of hydrocortisone

6. 0.9 g of sodium chloride are dissolved in 100 ml of the infusion
   9 g of sodium chloride are dissolved in 1 litre of the infusion
   58.5 g of sodium chloride is the weight of 1 mol or 1000 mmol
   1 g of sodium chloride is the weight of 1000 ÷ 58.5 mmol
   9 g of sodium chloride is the weight of (1000 ÷ 58.5) × 9 mmol = 153.8 mmol

7. 1 g of adrenaline is dissolved in 20,000 ml of solution
   1 mg of adrenaline is dissolved in 20,000 ÷ 1000 ml of solution = 20 ml
   50 mg of adrenaline is dissolved in 20 × 50 ml = 1000 ml = 1 litre

8. 1 mol of sodium bicarbonate weighs 84 g
   1000 mmol of sodium bicarbonate weighs 84 g
   Hence in the solution, 84 g of sodium bicarbonate are dissolved in 1000 ml
   Therefore 8.4 g are dissolved in 100 ml of the solution
   So, the concentration of the solution is 8.4% w/v

9. 1 g of the antiseptic is dissolved in 8000 ml of the solution
   1 ÷ 8000 g of the antiseptic is dissolved in 1 ml of the solution
   (1 ÷ 8000) × 200 g of the antiseptic is dissolved in 200 ml of the solution
   So, daily the patient uses (1 ÷ 8000) × 200 g of the antiseptic = 0.025 g
   In one week, the patient uses 0.025 g × 7 = 0.175 g of the antiseptic

10. First, we must calculate how much anhydrous drug is required to prepare the solution.

    4 g of the anhydrous drug must be dissolved in 100 ml of solution

4 ÷ 100 g of the anhydrous drug must be dissolved in 1 ml of solution

(4 ÷ 100) × 5000 g of the anhydrous drug must be dissolved in 5000 ml of solution = 200 g of anhydrous drug required

However, the drug powder contains 5% w/w moisture, therefore 95% w/w of the powder is the anhydrous drug

200 g of the anhydrous drug represents 95% of the weight of the powder required

Therefore the total weight of powder required = (200 ÷ 95) × 100 g = 210.5 g

Chapter 3

1. Prepare 250 ml of Acid Gentian Mixture BP

Concentrated compound gentian infusion	100 ml	25 ml
Dilute hydrochloric acid	50 ml	12.5 ml
Double strength chloroform water	500 ml	125 ml
Water	to 1000 ml	to 250 ml

2. Prepare 150 ml of Potassium Citrate Mixture BP

Potassium citrate	300 g	45 g
Citric acid monohydrate	50 g	7.5 g
Lemon spirit	5 ml	0.75 ml
Quillaia tincture	10 ml	1.5 ml
Syrup	250 ml	37.5 ml
Double strength chloroform water	300 ml	45 ml
Water	to 1000 ml	to 150 ml

3. Prepare 300 ml of Chloral Elixir Paed. BP

Chloral hydrate	200 mg	12 g
Water	0.1 ml	6 ml
Blackcurrant syrup	1 ml	60 ml
Syrup	to 5 ml	to 300 ml

4. Prepare 200 ml of Paediatric Ferrous Sulphate Mixture BP

Ferrous sulphate	60 mg	2.4 g
Ascorbic acid	10 mg	400 mg
Orange syrup	0.5 ml	20 ml
Double strength chloroform water	2.5 ml	100 ml
Water	to 5 ml	to 200 ml

5. What quantities of each ingredient are required to prepare 50 g of Coal Tar and Zinc Ointment BP?

Strong coal tar solution	100 g	5 g
Zinc oxide	300 g	15 g
Yellow soft paraffin	600 g	30 g

6. What quantity of each ingredient is required to prepare 600 g of Zinc and Salicylic acid Paste BP?

Zinc oxide	24%	144 g
Salicylic acid	2%	12 g
Starch	24%	144 g
White soft paraffin	50%	300 g

7. Prepare 5000 ml of Magnesium Hydroxide Mixture BP

Magnesium sulphate	47.5 g	237.5 g
Sodium hydroxide	15 g	75 g
Light Magnesium Oxide	52.5 g	262.5 g
Chloroform	2.5 ml	12.5 ml
Water	to 1000 ml	to 5000 ml

8. Prepare 30 g of the following ointment

Fluocinolone acetonide cream	10%	3 g
Aqueous cream	to 100%	to 30 g (i.e. 27 g)

9. Prepare 75 g of the following cream

Betamethasone cream	1 part	15 g
Aqueous cream	4 parts	60 g

10. Prepare 80 g of the following ointment

Dithranol ointment	1 part	20 g
White soft paraffin	to 4 parts	to 80 g (i.e. 60 g)

(*Note:* The second line of this formula states 'to 4 parts', indicating that white soft paraffin must comprise three parts of the ointment.)

Chapter 4

1. Use the formula $C_1 \times V_1 = C_2 \times V_2$

$C_1 = 0.2\%$ w/v
$V_1 = ?$
C_2 is a 1:5000 solution $= 0.02\%$ w/v
$V_2 = 1$ litre $= 1000$ ml
$0.2 \times V_1 = 0.02 \times 1000$
$V_1 = (0.02 \times 1000) \div 0.2 = 100$ ml

2. Again, use $C_1 \times V_1 = C_2 \times V_2$

    $C_1 = 4\%$ w/v
    $V_1 = 100$ ml
    C_2 is a 1:5000 solution $= 0.02\%$ w/v
    $V_2 = ?$
    $4 \times 100 = 0.02 \times V_2$
    $V_2 = (4 \times 100) \div 0.02 = 20,000$ ml $= 20$ litres

3. Determine what volume of the dilute solution the patient requires
    Daily the patient uses 50 ml $\times 2 = 100$ ml
    In five days, the patient uses 100 ml $\times 5 = 500$ ml

    Now use $C_1 \times V_1 = C_2 \times V_2$
    $C_1 = 2\%$ w/v
    $V_1 = ?$
    C_2 is a 1:10,000 solution of potassium permanganate $= 0.01\%$ w/v
    $V_2 = 500$ ml
    $2 \times V_1 = 0.01 \times 500$
    $V_1 = (0.01 \times 500) \div 2 = 2.5$ ml

4. $C_1 \times V_1 = C_2 \times V_2$
    $C_1 = 13\%$ w/v
    $V_1 = 50$ ml
    $C_2 = 0.65\%$ w/v
    $V_2 = ?$

    $13 \times 50 = 0.65 \times V_2$
    $V_2 = (13 \times 50) \div 0.65 = 1000$ ml

    Therefore to carry out the dilution, we must *add* 950 ml to the solution

5. Use $C_1 \times M_1 = C_2 \times M_2$
    $C_1 = 5\%$ w/w
    $M_1 = 200$ g
    $C_2 = 2\%$ w/w
    $M_2 = ?$

$5 \times 200 = 2 \times M_2$

$M_2 = (5 \times 200) \div 2 = 500\,g$

Therefore to carry out the dilution, we must add $500 - 200 = 300\,g$ of emulsifying ointment

6. $\dfrac{\text{Initial weight of drug} + \text{added weight of drug}}{\text{Initial volume of solution} + \text{added volume of solution}} = \dfrac{5}{100}$

$$\dfrac{0+x}{1000+\dfrac{100x}{25}} = \dfrac{5}{100}$$

$5000 + 20x = 100x$

$5000 = 80x$

$x = 62.5\,g$

62.5 g of dextrose are dissolved in $(100 \times 62.5) \div 25\,ml$ of the 25% w/v solution = 250 ml

7. The final concentration required is 40 mmol/l

1 mol of potassium weighs 39 g

1 mmol of potassium weighs $39 \div 1000\,g$

40 mmol of potassium weighs $(39 \div 1000) \times 40\,g = 1.56\,g$

Therefore the final concentration required is 1.56 g/l, or 0.156 g/100 ml = 0.156% w/v potassium chloride

$\dfrac{\text{Initial weight of drug} + \text{added weight of drug}}{\text{Initial volume of solution} + \text{added volume of solution}} = \dfrac{0.156}{100}$

Initial weight of drug = 0 g

Added weight of drug = x g

Initial volume of solution = 500 ml

Added volume of solution = $(100 \div 15)x$ g

$$\dfrac{0+x}{500+\dfrac{100x}{15}} = \dfrac{0.156}{100}$$

$100x = 78+x$

$99x = 78$

$x = 0.79\,g$

This weight of potassium chloride is dissolved in $(100 \div 15) \times 0.79\,ml = 5.27\,ml$

Therefore 5.27 ml of the potassium chloride solution should be added to the bag.

8. $$\frac{\text{Initial weight of drug} + \text{added weight of drug}}{\text{Initial weight of cream} + \text{added weight of drug}} = \frac{1}{100}$$

Initial weight of drug = 0.03 g (since we have 30 g of a 0.1% w/w cream)
Added weight of drug = x g
Initial weight of cream = 30 g

$$\frac{0.03 + x}{30 + x} = \frac{1}{100}$$

$100(0.03 + x) = 30 + x$
$3 + 100x = 30 + x$
$99x = 27$
$x = 0.27$ g

9. Use the same formula as the previous question

Initial weight of drug = 1 g (as we have 50 g of a 2% w/w ointment)
Added weight of drug = x g
Initial weight of ointment = 50 g

$$\frac{1 + x}{50 + x} = \frac{10}{100}$$

$100(1 + x) = 10(50 + x)$
$100 + 100x = 500 + 10x$
$90x = 400$
$x = 4.44$ g

10. The same formula can be used here as in the previous two questions – however, the unknown quantities are different. The initial weight of the 10% w/w ointment is unknown, but this must be made up to 30 g with the active ingredient.

Let the initial weight of the cream = x g
Initial weight of drug = $x/10$ g, or 0.1x g (since the initial cream contains 10% w/w coal tar solution)
Added weight of drug = (30 − x) g (since the final weight of the cream is 30 g)
Substituting into the equation

$$\frac{0.1x + (30 - x)}{x + (30 - x)} = \frac{12}{100}$$

Thus:

$$\frac{30 - 0.9x}{30} = \frac{12}{100}$$

$$100(30 - 0.9x) = 360$$
$$3000 - 90x = 360$$
$$90x = 2640$$
$$x = 29.33\,\text{g}$$

Therefore the initial weight of cream to be used = 29.33 g and 0.66 g of coal tar solution must be added to produce 30 g of a 12% w/w ointment.

Chapter 5

1. (a) Based on actual body weight, the dose required is 80 × 3 = 240 mg (rounded to the most convenient dose units, so that the prescription would be 250 mg daily).
   (b) Based on ideal body weight (IBW):

      IBW = (0.9 × 150) − 92 = 43 kg
      Total dose of phenytoin required = 43 × 3 = 129 mg
      Prescription would be 125 mg daily

2. Using the percentage method, since there is no quoted paediatric dose for drug x. From the table an average-weight two-month-old child could receive 15% of the adult dose. The adult dose for drug x is 600 mg, therefore the child could be prescribed a dose of 0.15 × 600 mg = 90 mg.

3. Using the equation in Chapter 5

$$\text{BSA} = \sqrt{\frac{H \times W}{3600}} = \sqrt{\frac{170 \times 65}{3600}} = 1.75\,\text{m}^2$$

Therefore the dose = 500 × 1.75 = 875 mg

4. (a) The syringe prepared contains 50 ml of 1000 U/ml. Prescription is for 2000 U/h, therefore the syringe rate must be 2 ml/h (2000 U/h ÷ 1000 U/ml).

   (b) If the total syringe volume is 50 ml and the rate is 2 ml/h
       the syringe will, theoretically, empty in 25 h (50/2).
          In practice, the syringe will not last the full 25 h since
       some its volume will be used to prime the line from the
       pump to the patient.

5. (a) Minimum administration time is 250 ÷ 4 = 62.5 min.
   (b) 250 mg frusemide are dissolved in 50 ml normal saline
       giving a concentration of 5 mg/ml (250 ÷ 50) and should be
       administered no more rapidly than 4 mg/min ÷ 5 mg/ml =
       0.8 ml/min.

6. Potassium concentration to be given is 80 mmol in 2 litre (i.e.
   40 mmol/l of fluid). The maximum speed at which this can be
   safely administered is 20 mmol/h and there are 20 mmol of
   potassium in 500 ml of fluid at this concentration. Therefore the
   maximum rate at which the fluid can be administered is
   500 ml/h or 8.3 ml/min (500 ÷ 60). Since there are 20 drops per
   millilitre for this giving set, the maximum drip rate is 20 × 8.3 =
   166 drops per minute.

7. The number of drops that will be provided from 250 ml will be
   250 × 60 = 15,000. There are 24 × 60 min in 24 h = 1440 min.
   Therefore the drop rate should be 15,000 drops ÷ 1440 min =
   10.4 drops/min.

8. The concentration of insulin in the pump is 75 U in 50 ml saline
   or 1.5 U/ml. The patient's blood glucose is currently 12.3 mmol
   and from the table this corresponds to an insulin dose of 3 U/h.
   The resulting pump rate should therefore be 3 U/h ÷ 1.5 U/ml =
   2 ml/h.

9. The concentration of dopamine in the syringe is 4 mg/ml
   (200 ÷ 50). The pump is running at 3.1 ml/h delivering a total
   of 12.4 mg/h, which corresponds to 206.67 mcg/min
   (12.4 × 1000) ÷ 60, giving a dose of 2.95 mcg/kg/min or
   (rounding up) 3 mcg/kg/min (206.67 ÷ 70).

10. The concentration of dobutamine in the syringe is 250 mg in
    50 ml or 5 mg/ml (250 ÷ 50). The current pump rate is 2.4 ml/h
    or 12 mg/h (2.4 × 5), which is 0.2 mg/min or 200 mcg/min. This
    corresponds to a dose of 3 mcg/kg/min (200/65). Increasing this
    dose by 0.5 mcg/kg/min gives 3.5 mcg/kg/min, or
    227.5 mcg/min (3.5 × 65), or 13.65 mg/h ((227.5 × 60) ÷ 1000),
    which gives a pump rate of 2.7 ml/h (13.65 ÷ 5) and an
    increase in pump rate of 0.3 ml/h (2.7 − 2.4).

Chapter 6

1. Bioavailability F = 1
   Salt fraction S = 1

$$\text{Volume of Distribution} = \frac{F \times S \times \text{Dose}}{C}$$

$$= \frac{1 \times 1 \times 1200 \text{ mg}}{12 \text{ mg}/l}$$

$$= 100 \text{ litres}$$

2. Amount of drug reaching systemic circulation = Bioavailability × Salt fraction × Dose administered

$$= F \times S \times \text{Dose}$$

Assuming that the amount excreted in the urine represents the amount systemically absorbed, then:

$85 \text{ mcg} = F \times 1 \times 100 \text{ mcg}$
Hence $F = 0.85$

3. From previous information, the $T_{0.5}$ for theophylline = 8 h. Therefore the time taken for the serum concentration to fall to one-quarter of its original value will be 16 h.

4. IBW (male) = $0.9H - 88 = (0.9 \times 165 \text{ cm}) - 92 = 56.5 \text{ kg}$. The weight used in the equation is therefore 55 kg:

$$Cl_{cr} = \frac{1.23(140 - \text{Age}) \times \text{Weight (kg)}}{\text{Serum creatinine } (\mu mol/litre)}$$

$$= \frac{1.23(140 - 80) \times 55}{180}$$

$$= 22.5 \text{ ml/min (mild renal impairment)}$$

5. Bioavailability F $= 1$
   Salt fraction S $= 1$
   Volume of distribution V_d $= 7.3$ litre/kg
   Target concentration $= 1.5$ mcg/l

This patient's volume of distribution is therefore

$$7.3 \text{ l/kg} \times 60 \text{ kg} = 438 \text{ litre}$$

$$= \frac{V_d \times C}{F \times S}$$

$$= \frac{438 \, \text{litre} \times 1.5 \, \text{mcg}/l}{1 \times 1}$$

$$= 657 \, \text{mcg digoxin tablets}$$
$$(687.5 \, \text{mcg in practice})$$

6. Bioavailability F = 1
   Salt fraction S = 0.8
   Volume of distribution V_d = 0.5 litre/kg
   Target concentration   = 10 mg/l

This patient's volume of distribution is therefore

$$0.5 \, \text{litre/kg} \times 65 \, \text{kg} = 32.5 \, \text{litre}$$

$$\text{Required dose} = \frac{\text{Volume of distribution } (V_d) \times \text{Concentration } (C)}{\text{Bioavailability } (F) \times \text{Salt fraction } (S)}$$

$$= 406.2 \, \text{mg aminophylline}$$

7. Bioavailability F = 1
   Salt fraction S = 1
   Volume of distribution V_d = 0.25 litre/kg

This patient's volume of distribution is therefore

$$0.25 \, \text{litre/kg} \times 70 \, \text{kg} = 17.5 \, \text{litre}$$

To estimate the concentration, the equation for determining loading dosages:

$$\text{Required dose} = \frac{\text{Volume of distribution } (V_d) \times \text{Concentration } (C)}{\text{Bioavailability } (F) \times \text{Salt fraction } (S)}$$

needs to be rearranged, as follows:

$$C = \frac{\text{Dose} \times F \times S}{V_d}$$

$$= \frac{100 \, \text{mg} \times 1 \times 1}{17.5 \, \text{litre}}$$

$$= 5.71 \, \text{mg/l}$$

8. Bioavailability F = 0.7 for digoxin tablets
   Salt fraction S = 1
   Desired serum concentration C = 1.5 mcg/l

Firstly we need to calculate the ideal body weight:

IBW (female) = $0.9H - 92 = 0.9(160) - 92 = 52 \, \text{kg}$
In this case the weight to be used is the IBW. Next we need to determine the patient's renal function:

$$Cl_{cr} = \frac{1.04 \, (140 - \text{Age}) \times \text{Weight (kg)}}{\text{Serum creatinine (}\mu\text{mol/l)}}$$

$$Cl_{cr} \, (\text{females}) = \frac{1.04 \, (140 - 75) \times 52}{170}$$

Therefore Cl_{cr} = 20.7 ml/min (mild renal impairment)

Next we need to determine the digoxin clearance for a patient with congestive heart failure:

Digoxin clearance (ml/min) = $(0.33 \times \text{Weight (kg)}) + (0.9 \times Cl_{cr})$
= $(0.33 \times 52) + (0.9 \times 20.7)$
= $17.2 + 18.60 = 35.8 \, \text{ml/min}$
= $2.15 \, \text{litre/h}$

Finally, we can calculate the recommended maintenance dose:

$$\text{Maintenance dose} = \frac{\text{Clearance (litre/h)} \times \text{Concentration (mg/l)} \times \tau}{\text{Bioavailability } (F) \times \text{Salt fraction } (S)}$$

$$= \frac{2.15 \times 1.5 \times 24}{0.7 \times 1}$$

= 110.6 mcg daily (125 mcg in practice)

9. Bioavailability F = 1
   Salt fraction S = 0.92
   K_m = 4 mg/l

Firstly, we need to calculate V_m:

$$V_{\mathrm{m}} = \frac{S \times F \times \text{Daily dose (mg)} \times (K_{\mathrm{m}} + \text{Serum concentration})}{\text{Serum concentration}}$$

$$= \frac{0.92 \times 1 \times 300 \times (4 + 8)}{8}$$

$$= 414 \, \text{mg/day}$$

$$\text{Daily dose (mg)} = \frac{V_{\mathrm{m}} \times \text{Serum concentration}}{S \times F \times (K_{\mathrm{m}} + \text{Serum concentration})}$$

$$= \frac{414 \times 12}{1 \times 0.92 \times (4 + 12)}$$

= 337.5 mg phenytoin sodium capsules (350 mg in practice)

10. $F = 0.85$
$S = 1$
$C = 10 \, \text{mg/l}$
$\tau = 12 \, \text{h}$
$V_{\mathrm{d}} = 0.064 \, \text{litre/h/kg}$

Patient's clearance of carbamazepine = 0.064 litre/h/kg × 70 kg

$$= 4.48 \, \text{litre/h}$$

$$\text{Maintenance dose} = \frac{\text{Clearance (litre/h)} \times \text{Concentration (mg/l)} \times \tau}{\text{Bioavailability } (F) \times \text{Salt fraction } (S)}$$

$$= \frac{4.48 \times 10 \times 12}{0.85 \times 1}$$

= 632 mg every 12 h (600 mg 12-hourly in practice)

Chapter 7

1. Total weight of the suppositories = 14 g
Weight of the drug required (2.5% w/w) = (14 × 2.5) ÷ 100 = 0.35 g
Therefore the weight of base required = 14 g − 0.35 g = 13.65 g

2. Total weight of the suppositories = 12 g
   Weight of the drug required = (12 × 10) ÷ 100 = 1.2 g
   Therefore the weight of base required = 12 – 1.2 g = 10.8 g

3. Total weight of medicament required = 6 × 125 mg = 750 mg =
   0.75 g
   Weight of base for six unmedicated suppositories = 6 × 2 g =
   12 g
   As the displacement value of paracetamol = 1.5,
   1.5 g of paracetamol will displace 1 g of theobroma oil,
   1 g of paracetamol will displace 1 ÷ 1.5 g of theobroma oil
   Therefore 0.75 g of paracetamol will displace 0.75 ÷ 1.5 g of
   theobroma oil = 0.5 g
   Therefore the weight of base required to make medicated
   suppositories = 12 g – 0.5 g = 11.5 g

4. Total weight of aspirin required = 12 × 300 mg = 3600 mg =
   3.6 g
   Weight of base required for unmedicated suppositories =
   12 × 2 g = 24 g
   As the displacement value of aspirin = 1.1,
   1.1 g of aspirin will displace 1 g of theobroma oil,
   1 g of aspirin will displace 1 ÷ 1.1 g of theobroma oil
   Therefore 3.6 g of aspirin will displace (1 × 3.6) ÷ 1.1 g of theobroma oil = 3.27 g of theobroma oil
   Therefore the weight of base required required to make medicated suppositories = 24 g – 3.27 g = 20.73 g

5. Weight of bismuth subgallate required = 10 × 50 mg = 500 mg
   or 0.5 g
   Weight of base required for unmedicated suppositories =
   10 × 2 g = 20 g
   As the displacement value of bismuth subgallate = 2.7,
   2.7 g of bismuth subgallate will displace 1 g of theobroma oil,
   1 g of bismuth subgallate will displace 1 ÷ 2.7 g of theobroma oil
   0.5 g of bismuth subgallate will displace (1 × 0.5) ÷ 2.7 g of
   theobroma oil = 0.18 g
   Therefore the weight of base required to make medicated
   suppositories = 20 g – 0.18 g = 19.82 g

6. Total weight of the suppositories = 8 × 4 g × 1.2 = 38.4 g
   Weight of hydrocortisone acetate required = (38.4 g × 1) ÷
   100 = 0.384 g
   Therefore the weight of the base required = 38.4 g – 0.384 g =
   38.016 g

7. Total weight of morphine hydrochloride required = 6 × 20 mg =
   120 mg = 0.12 g

Weight of base required for unmedicated suppositories = 6 × 2 g × 1.2 = 14.4 g

As the displacement value of morphine hydrochloride = 1.6,

1.6 g of morphine hydrate displaces 1 g of theobroma oil,

1 g of morphine hydrate displaces 1 ÷ 1.6 g of theobroma oil

and 0.12 g of morphine hydrate displaces (1 × 0.12) ÷ 1.6 g of theobroma oil = 0.075 g of theobroma oil

This means that the drug will displace 0.075 g × 1.2 of the glycero-gelatin base = 0.09 g

Therefore the weight of base required to make medicated suppositories = 14.4 g – 0.09 g = 14.31 g

8. Total weight of phenobarbitone sodium required = 10 × 30 mg = 300 mg = 0.3 g

Total weight of unmedicated suppositories = 10 × 1 g × 1.2 = 12 g

As the displacement value of phenobarbitone sodium = 1.2,

1.2 g of phenobarbitone sodium will displace 1 g of theobroma oil,

1 g of phenobarbitone sodium will displace 1 ÷ 1.2 g of theobroma oil,

and 0.3 g of phenobarbitone sodium will displace (1 × 0.3) ÷ 1.2 g of theobroma oil = 0.25 g of theobroma oil

This means that the drug will displace 0.25 g × 1.2 of the glycero-gelatin base = 0.3 g

Therefore the weight of base required to make medicated suppositories = 12 g – 0.3 g = 11.7 g

9. Total weight of diphenhydramine hydrochloride required = 12 × 50 mg = 600 mg = 0.6 g

Total weight of unmedicated suppositories = 12 × 2 g × 1.2 = 28.8 g

As the displacement value of diphenhydramine hydrochloride = 1.3,

1.3 g of diphenhydramine hydrochloride will displace 1 g of theobroma oil,

1 g of diphenhydramine hydrochloride will displace 1 ÷ 1.3 g of theobroma oil

0.6 g of diphenhydramine hydrochloride will displace (1 × 0.6) ÷ 1.3 g of theobroma oil = 0.46 g

This means that the drug will displace 0.46 g × 1.2 of glycero-gelatin base = 0.55 g

Therefore the weight of base required to make medicated suppositories = 28.8 g – 0.55 g = 28.25 g

10. Total weight of bismuth subgallate required = 10 × 60 mg = 600 mg = 0.6 g

Total weight of hydrocortisone acetate required = 10 × 10 mg = 100 mg = 0.1 g

Total weight of unmedicated suppositories = 10 × 2 g = 20 g

As the displacement value of bismuth subgallate = 2.7,

2.7 g of bismuth subgallate will displace 1 g of theobroma oil,

1 g of bismuth subgallate will displace 1 ÷ 2.7 g of theobroma oil
0.6 g of bismuth subgallate will displace (1 × 0.6) ÷ 2.7 g of theobroma oil = 0.22 g of theobroma oil

As the displacement value of hydrocortisone acetate = 1.5,

1.5 g of hydrocortisone acetate will displace 1 g of theobroma oil,

1 g of hydrocortisone acetate will displace 1 ÷ 1.5 g of theobroma oil

0.1 g of hydrocortisone acetate will displace (1 × 0.1) ÷ 1.5 g of theobroma oil = 0.15 g of theobroma oil

Total weight of theobroma oil displaced = 0.22 g + 0.15 g = 0.37 g

Therefore the weight of base required to make medicated suppositories = 20 g − 0.37 g = 19.63 g

Answers to the Summary Test

1. 0.25 litre =   250 ml
   75 ml =   75 ml
   4000 µl =   4 ml

   Total volume = 329 ml

2. Daily, the patient must take 5 ml × 4 = 20 ml
   In seven days the patient will take 20 ml × 7 = 140 ml

3. 1 mol of potassium chloride weighs 74.5 g
   Therefore 1 mmol of potassium chloride weighs 74.5 mg
   So, 80 mmol of potassium chloride weighs 74.5 × 80 mg = 5960 mg or 5.96 g

4. 100 g of the cream contains 2 g of salicylic acid
   1 g of the cream contains 2/100 g of salicylic acid
   350 g of the cream contains 2 × 350/100 g of salicylic acid = 7 g of salicylic acid

5. 1 g of adrenaline is dissolved in 10,000 ml of the solution
   1 mg of adrenaline is dissolved in 10 ml of the solution (10,000/1,000)
   20 mg of adrenaline is dissolved in 200 ml of the solution

6. 1 g of antiseptic is dissolved in 1000 ml of the mouthwash
   1/1000 g of antiseptic is dissolved in 1 ml of the mouthwash
   50/1000 g of antiseptic is dissolved in 50 ml of the mouthwash = 0.05 g
   Daily, the patient uses 0.05 g × 4 of the antiseptic = 0.2 g
   In seven days, the patient uses 0.2 g × 7 of the antiseptic = 1.4 g

7. Chloral Elixir Paed. BP

Chloral hydrate	200 mg	20 g
Water	0.1 ml	10 ml
Blackcurrant syrup	1 ml	100 ml
Syrup	to 5 ml	to 500 ml

8. Coal Tar and Zinc Ointment BP

Strong coal tar solution	100 g	15 g
Zinc oxide	300 g	45 g
Yellow soft paraffin	600 g	90 g
Total weight	1000 g	150 g

9. Zinc and Salicylic acid Paste BP

Zinc oxide	24%	96 g
Salicylic acid	2%	8 g
Starch	24%	96 g
White soft paraffin	50%	200 g
Total weight	400 g	

10. For the 1:10,000 solution:

1 g of potassium permanganate is dissolved in 10,000 ml of the solution

0.01 g of potassium permanganate is dissolved in 100 ml of the solution

Therefore the patient is using a 0.01% w/v solution of potassium permanganate

Daily, the patient uses 20 ml × 2 = 40 ml

In 10 days the patient uses 40 ml × 10 = 400 ml

Now apply the dilution formula $C_1 \times V_1 = C_2 \times V_2$:

$C_1 = 4\%$ w/v
$V_1 = ?$
C_2 is a 1:10,000 solution of potassium permanganate = 0.01% w/v
$V_2 = 400$ ml

$4 \times V_1 = 0.01 \times 400$
$4 \times V_1 = 4$
$V_1 = 1$ ml

11. Use $C_1 \times M_1 = C_2 \times M_2$:

$C_1 = 2\%$ w/w
$M_1 = 400$ g
$C_2 = 0.5\%$ w/w
$M_2 = ?$

$2 \times 400 = 0.5 \times M_2$

Therefore $M_2 = 1600\,g$

Hence in order to carry out the dilution, we must add $1600 - 400 = 1200\,g$ of emulsifying ointment.

12. $$\frac{\text{Initial weight of drug} + \text{added weight of drug}}{\text{Initial volume of solution} + \text{added volume of solution}} = \frac{4}{100}$$

$$\frac{0 + x}{500 + \dfrac{100x}{40}} = \frac{4}{100}$$

$$2000 + 10x = 100x$$
$$2000 = 90x$$
$$x = 22.2\,g$$

22.2 g of dextrose are dissolved in $(100 \times 22.2) \div 40\,ml$ of the 40% w/v solution = 55.5 ml

13. $$\frac{\text{Initial weight of drug} + \text{added weight of drug}}{\text{Initial weight of cream} + \text{added weight of drug}} = \frac{5}{100}$$

Initial weight of drug = 2 g (since we have 200 g of a 1% w/w cream)
Added weight of drug = x g
Initial weight of cream = 200 g

$$\frac{2 + x}{200 + x} = \frac{5}{100}$$

$$1000 + 5x = 200 + 100x$$
$$800 = 95x$$
$$x = 8.42\,g$$

14. Firstly we need to determine the concentration per millilitre of the bumetanide in the glucose 5% w/v solution. 5 mg in 500 ml = 5000 mcg in 500 ml = 10 mcg/ml. If the maximum rate is 100 mcg/min and 100 mcg can be found in 10 ml of solution, then the maximum rate will be 10 ml/min.

15. Determine the amount of dopamine administered over 1 h. If there is 160 mg/50 ml in the original solution and the infusion rate is 5 ml/h, then the patient is receiving 16 mg/h. They are therefore receiving 16 mg/h which is 0.267 mg/min =

267 mcg/min. If the patient weighs 80 kg then they are receiving 267/80 mcg/kg/min = 3.3 mcg/kg/min.

16. Firstly we need to calculate the patient's ideal body weight (IBW):

    IBW (female) = $0.9H - 92 = (0.9 \times 170\,cm) - 92 = 61\,kg$
    Therefore ABW is lower.

    The equation for calculating renal function is:

    $$Cl_{cr}\ (females) = \frac{1.04(140 - Age) \times Weight\ (kg)}{Serum\ creatinine\ (\mu mol\,/\,l)}\ ml\,/\,min$$

    $$= \frac{1.04(140 - 80) \times 60}{170\,\mu mol\,/\,l)}\ ml\,/\,min$$

    $$= 22.2\,ml/min$$

    We can therefore assume that this patient has mild renal impairment.

17. Determine the patient's ideal body weight (IBW):

    Males   IBW = $(0.9 \times H) - 88 = 74\,kg$

    Therefore the IBW is lower than the ABW.

    From Chapter 6, bioavailability of digoxin $F = 0.7$, salt fraction $S = 1$ and volume of distribution per kilogram of lean body weight is $V_d/kg = 7.3$ litre/kg.
    From the question the target concentration C is 1.2 mcg/l.

    $$Loading\ dose = \frac{C \times V_d}{F \times S}$$

    $$\frac{1.2\ mg\,/\,l \times 7.3\,litre\,/\,kg \times 74\,kg}{0.7 \times 1} = 926\ mcg$$

    Hence either 937.5 mcg or 1000 mcg could be prescribed.

18. From the last question, the patient's IBW was calculated to be 74 kg. We know from Chapter 6 that $F = 0.7$ for digoxin tablets, $S = 1$, from the question the target concentration $C = 1.2$ mcg/l,

renal function Cl_{cr} = 18 ml/min and dosage interval τ = 24 h. Firstly, we need to determine the digoxin clearance for a patient with congestive heart failure. From Chapter 6:

$$
\begin{aligned}
\text{Digoxin clearance (ml/min)} &= 0.33 \times \text{Weight (kg)} + 0.9Cl_{cr} \\
&= (0.33 \times 74\,\text{kg}) + (0.9 \times 18\,\text{ml/min}) \\
&= 40.6\,\text{ml/min} \\
&= 2.4\,\text{litre/h}
\end{aligned}
$$

Finally, we can calculate the recommended maintenance dose:

$$
\text{Maintenance dose} = \frac{\text{Digoxin clearance } (\ell/\text{h}) \times \text{Concentration (mcg/l)} \times \tau}{\text{Bioavailability } (F) \times \text{Salt fraction } (S)}
$$

$$
= \frac{2.4\,\text{litre/h} \times 1.2\,\text{mcg/l} \times 24\,\text{h}}{0.7 \times 1}
$$

$$
= 98\,\text{mcg daily}
$$

Either 62.5 mcg or 125 mcg could be prescribed on a daily basis.

19. Weight of bismuth subgallate required = $12 \times 100\,\text{mg}$ = 1.2 g

    Weight of base required for unmedicated suppositories = $12 \times 4\,\text{g}$ = 48 g
    As the displacement value of bismuth subgallate = 2.7,
    2.7 g of bismuth subgallate will displace 1 g of theobroma oil,
    1 g of bismuth subgallate will displace $1 \div 2.7$ g of theobroma oil,
    1.2 g of bismuth subgallate will displace $(1 \times 1.2) \div 2.7$ g of theobroma oil = 0.44 g
    Therefore weight of base required to make medicated suppositories = 48 g − 0.44 g = 47.56 g

20. Total weight of the suppositories = $6 \times 2\,\text{g} \times 1.2$ = 14.4 g
    Weight of hydrocortisone acetate required = $(14.4\,\text{g} \times 0.5) \div 100$ = 0.07 g
    Therefore weight of the base required = 14.4 g − 0.07 g = 14.33 g

7. Estimate the maximum serum concentration of a 70 kg patient that would be expected, after a loading dose of 480 mg have been given (assuming that a test dose had been negligible concentration after)?

8. What daily maintenance dose of digoxin would you recommend for a 65-year-old, 55 kg female (5 ft tall) with congestive heart failure and a measured serum creatinine of 120 µmol/l?

9. A 75 kg patient prescribed 300 mg of phenytoin capsules daily has a measured serum concentration of 8 mg/l. What dosage of phenytoin would you recommend in order to obtain a serum concentration of 12 mg/l?

10. What twice-daily maintenance dose of carbamazepine (slow release tablets) would you recommend for a 70 kg male, if the target concentration was 10 mg/l?

7 Suppository Calculations

By the end of this chapter you should be able to:

* calculate quantities of base and drug required for the preparation of theobroma oil and glycerol-gelatin based suppositories

7.1 Suppositories

Suppositories are dosage forms prepared for drug delivery via the rectum. These consist of an active medicament dispersed throughout an inactive base. The bases used in these products can be broadly classified into two groups:

* Fatty bases. These may be of natural origin, such as theobroma oil (cocoa butter), or synthetic fats such as Witepsol.
* Hydrophilic bases. The most commonly used hydrophilic base is composed of a solid glycerol-gelatin mixture.

Displacement Values

Suppositories are prepared by dissolving or dispersing an active medicament in a molten base and pouring the mixture into a suppository mould. Suppository moulds are normally available in 1 g, 2 g and 4 g sizes – the approximate weights of the theobroma oil suppositories that are produced from them – although the volume of the suppository mould will be constant. However, because the density of the medicament may vary considerably from that of the base, the weight of the base required to make a suppository will vary depending on the medicament used. For example, 2 g of a medicament with twice the density of theobroma oil would occupy approximately the same volume as 1 g of the suppository base. The displacement values (DVs) of